SUPREET KAUR
SAVREEN KAUR
GURPREET SINGH

MIXED DENTITION ANALYSIS

SUPREET KAUR
SAVREEN KAUR
GURPREET SINGH

MIXED DENTITION ANALYSIS

LAP LAMBERT Academic Publishing

Imprint

Cover image: www.ingimage.com

Publisher:
LAP LAMBERT Academic Publishing
is a trademark of
Dodo Books Indian Ocean Ltd. and OmniScriptum S.R.L publishing group

120 High Road, East Finchley, London, N2 9ED, United Kingdom
Str. Armeneasca 28/1, office 1, Chisinau MD-2012, Republic of Moldova, Europe
Managing Directors: Ieva Konstantinova, Victoria Ursu
info@omniscriptum.com

Printed at: see last page
ISBN: 978-620-8-47236-8

INDEX

INTRODUCTION

Mixed dentition period is the most dynamic phase in terms of changes in occlusion and final outcome of dento-skeletal relationship. During the mixed dentition period, the orthodontist and pediatric dentist is often asked to provide an accurate diagnosis and treatment of any developing malocclusions. Early intervention of the developing malocclusions can be done by a proper space assessment in mixed dentition phase. Thus, mixed dentition arch analysis forms an essential part of diagnostic procedures.

Early treatment is becoming increasingly popular in the orthodontic circles and it is imperative that the mixed dentition space analysis is accurately done before such orthodontic treatment is offered[1]. Prominent among the conditions requiring early attention are those in which there is disparity between the amount of the dental arch space and the amount of tooth material, which should be accommodated. In planning the most expeditious management of such cases it is imperative that any deficit of arch space be predicted in advance and the indicated procedures instituted early[2].

An accurate mixed dentition space analysis is one of the important criteria in determining whether the treatment plan may involve serial extraction, guidance of eruption, space maintenance, space regaining or just periodic observation of the patients[3]. There have been instances in which space maintaining appliances were placed in areas where space was already grossly inadequate, with the result that tooth extraction was necessary along with orthodontic space closure of the very space which was held open. The consequence, of course, was a needless appliance, an unnecessary expense, and a protraction of orthodontic treatment[2].

Mixed dentition analysis involves a decision process whereby the space required for the dentition is subtracted from the space available within the arch. The space required is the sum of the total mesiodistal dimensions of the permanent canines and premolars on each side of the arch plus the width of the four permanent incisors. Space available is measured usually involve one of two methods. The first involves placing a brass wire through the contact points of each tooth, then measuring the length of the brass wire when straightened out. The second method, space available can be measured most easily by dividing the dental arch into 4 straight -line segments. Each segment is measured individually with a sharp pointed measuring instrument (dividers, a sharpened boley's guage). If space required is greater than space available then there is arch perimeter space deficiency, crowding would occur. If available space is larger than the space required then gaps between some teeth would be expected.[1]

Tooth size prediction of the unerupted permanent canines, first and second premolars forms part of the critical aspects of the mixed dentition space analysis. Three main approaches have been used to estimate the mesiodistal crown widths of the permanent canines and premolars in the mixed dentition patients:

1. Measurement of unerupted teeth on the radiographs (Nance, 1947[4]; Huckaba, 1964).
2. Use of the regression equations that relate the mesio-distal widths of erupted teeth to the mesio-distal widths of unerupted teeth (Moyers, 1958, 1973,1988; Tanaka and Johnson, 1974)[5]
3. A combination of measurements from erupted teeth and radiographs of unerupted teeth (Hixon and Oldfather, 1958[6];Foster and Wylie,1958)[7]

The most accurate predictons of the mesio-distal widths of unerupted canines and premolars can be obtained by measurements of mesio-distal widths of these teeth on radiographs combined with measurement of mesio-distal widths of the erupted mandibular permanent teeth [8].

Management of space problems continues to play an important role in a dental practice. Accurate prediction of mesiodistal width of unerupted permanent teeth is required to determine tooth size and arch length discrepancies in mixed dentition. Inaccurate mixed dentition space analysis may lead to wrong extraction decision and poor patient's facial profile. As patient's demand to seek an early orthodontic treatment is increasing therefore it is important for paedodontists to predict any discrepancy in arch space in advance and initiate appropriate treatment in a timely manner. [1]

REVIEW OF LITERATURE

Nance (1947)[4] The Nance analysis incorporates the summation of the lower central and lateral permanent incisors (as measured from the casts) with the sum of the unerupted lower canines and premolars found on the radiographs. This yields the total space required and is compared with the total space available, as measured directly from the casts. Nance further observed that in the average patient's mandibular arch a leeway of 1.7 mm per side exists between the combined mesiodistal widths of the primary mandibular canine and first and second primary molars and the mesiodistal widths of the corresponding permanent teeth, with the primary teeth being larger. This difference in the total mesiodistal width of the corresponding three primary teeth in the maxillary arch compared with the width of the three permanent teeth that succeed them is only 0.9 mm per side. He concluded that the distance from the mesiolingual of the mandibular first permanent molar to the mandibular midline likewise always shortens in the transition from the mixed to the permanent dentition. The total predicted arch length is what is important to orthodontists and pedodontists, In as much as that value aids in the decision as to whether or not to extract teeth

Ballard M.L. et al (1947)[9] studied the amount of harmony between groups of human mandibular teeth with respect to mesiodistal width and it is indicated by coefficients of correlation. From the coefficients of correlation they derived a predictive graph which makes it possible for one, knowing the sum of the mesiodistal widths of the four mandibular incisors to arrive at the total sum of the mesiodistal widths of the mandibular canine, first premolar, and second premolar of one side. The average error found to arise from the use of this predictive graph was 0.6 mm. or 2.6 per cent. In the same group of cases, using measurements taken from models of the permanent dentition as the correct values, the average error arising from the use of intraoral dental films of average quality taken in the mixed dentition was found to be 2.2 mm. or 10.5 per cent. The predictive graph will give only the sum of the unerupted teeth of one side in the mixed dentition, and does not provide an estimate of the mesiodistal width of any one of the three teeth. As such it is offered as an adjunct to the method of the mixed dentition diagnosis and ease analysis of Nance.

Seipel (1946)[10] attempted to predict the mesio-distal width of mandibular permanent canine and premolar teeth based on the mesio-distal width of the corresponding mandibular central incisor. The correlation coefficient was found to be low in all three cases. seipel measured the sizes of separate teeth, the position of the teeth, and orientation of the dentition to adjacent parts of the skull. Included were such measurements as transverse dimensions of the dental arch, length of the dental arch, and intermaxillary relations. These measurements were taken from three age groups: aged 4 years; aged 13 years; and aged 21 years. It was found that there is a. pronounced positive correlation with regard to the size of teeth in the same jaw with the different component varying in the same direction in relation to the mean value. Individuals with large incisors also have other teeth of larger than average size. He shows that while frequent positional variations of spacing and crowding appear in size-space, disturbances there are also specific from variations which appear independent of available space in the jaws.

Moorrees C.F.A. et al (1957)[11] investigated, by measurements on dental casts of 184 North American children of European ancestry, (91 males and 93 females) studied longitudinally from 3 to 18 years of age, the relationship between the mesio-distal crown widths of primary and permanent teeth. Impressions of the deciduous dentitions were made with modeling compound and those of the permanent dentitions with a hydrocolloid material. The correlation coefficient was low, reflecting great individual variation within the population. A sex difference was noted, males having larger teeth than females; therefore the results were analysed for males and females separately. They found that permanent incisor and canine teeth were larger than their predecessors, whereas premolar teeth were smaller. They concluded that measurement of unerupted permanent canines and premolars on radiographs was more accurate than estimation by measurement of the primary dentition.

Foster & Wylie (1958)[7]examined 72 children at 18- month intervals over a period of 10 years, 14 children being available at the end of the study. They found that the reduction in arch length was variable, but generally less than that reported by Nance. They also estimated the size of unerupted permanent canines and premolars by two methods: the Ballard & Wylie method, and by measuring the teeth on radiographs taken by the long-cone technique. They compared these estimates with the actual sizes of the teeth after they had erupted. Both methods showed inaccuracies, ranging from overestimates of 3.9 and 4.0 mm and underestimates of 5.7 and 1.6 mm by the Ballard & Wylie and radiographic methods, respectively.

Bolton (1958)[12] conducted a study on fifty five excellent occlusion cases and various measurements were made on casts. Three inch needle pointed dividers were used to determine the greatest mesiodistal diameter of all the teeth on each cast, excepting second and third molar. The dimensions to the nearest one-quarter millimeter were taken from a finely caliberated millimeter ruler and recorded. These measurements included determination of the mesiodistal diameters of all the individual teeth, certain buccal segment measurements, as well as, degree of overjet and overbite, the angle of the maxillary central incisor to the mandibular central incisor, central incisor lengths, the cusp height. He concluded that tooth size data was closely related to Black and Ballard. The statistical evaluation given by Ballard and Wylie in the study on mixed dentition case analysis was repeated in this investigation with very similar results.

Hixon & Oldfather (1958)[6] examined the dental casts and periapical radiographs of 41 children in the mixed dentition, and the casts of the same children taken following the eruption of canines and premolars. Utilizing a 16 inch target-film distance they found a weak correlation between the mesiodistal widths of the primary and permanent teeth. The correlation coefficient between the sum of the widths of mandibular permanent incisors and that of mandibular permanent canines and premolars, measured on the casts, was similar to that reported by other authors (0.69). The strongest correlation (0.88) was between, on the one hand, the sum of the widths of the central and lateral incisors in one quadrant, measured on the casts, added to the sum of the widths of the two premolars in the same quadrant, measured on radiographs, and, on the other, the sum of the widths of the canines and premolars after their eruption. From these results the authors devised a table for prediction of the mesio-distal widths of unerupted canines and premolars.

Tweed C.H. (1963)[13] The Tweed diagnostic facial triangle was concerned as a basis for diagnosis and treatment planning. It consists of:FMA – Frankfort mandibular plane angle, IMPA – Incisor mandibular plane angle ,FMIA – Frankfort mandibular incisor angle. Tweed Estd. 25^0 as normal for FMA, 90^0 for IMPA, 65^0 for FMIA. The value for space required and space available was assessed according to conventional method. The Tweed foundation research established the following relationships. When FMA is between 21^0 - 29^0 FMIA should be 68^0.When FMA is 30^0 or greater – FMIA = 65.^{0} When FMA is 20^0 or less – IMPA should not exceed 92.^{0}If the cephalometric tracing did not correspond to the above objectives, an objective line was traced to form the required FMIA. Then the distension between this and the line that passed through the actual axial inclination of mandibular incisors was measured on the occlusal plane. The figure is multiplied by 2 to include right and left sides. The total is the cephalometric correction which is added to the difference got by conventional method to give the total discrepancy.

Huckaba G.W. (1964)[4] He uses both study casts and radiographs for determining the width of un-erupted tooth using principle that with any type of radiograph, it is necessary to compensate for enlargement of the radiographic image. This can be done by measuring an object that can be seen both in radiograph and on the cast, such as primary molar tooth. Due to the possibility of radiographic elongation or shortening, the author recognized the need to compensate for radiographic distortion. He developed the procedure on the basis that the degree of magnification on a given film is approximately the same for a primary tooth as for its permanent successor. He also determined that the rnandibular permanent incisors were the most reliable indices of the size of the remaining permanent teeth of both arches. A simple proportional relationship can then be established as follows:

Actual width of primary molar (XI)

Apparent width of primary molar (X2)

Actual width of unerupted premolar (YI)

Apparent width of unerupted premolar (Y2)

$$YI = \frac{XI \times Y2}{X2}$$

Tanaka M.M. et al (1974)[5] used linear regression equations for the prediction of the mesiodistal widths of unerupted canines and premolars and calculated for a large sample of recent orthodontic patients. Dental casts for 506 orthodontic patients in the Cleveland area were obtained from the orthodontic department of Case Western Reserve University School of Dentistry and from the records of three orthodontists practicing in the Cleveland area, Drs. Sanford Neuger, Arthur Phelps, and Milton Rabine. To be included in the study, patients had to be of probable European ancestry and less than 20 years old. Models had to have been taken since 1966 before any orthodontic treatment, and all teeth to be measured had to be fully erupted and free of visible fractures, caries, and restorations. Mesiodistal width of permanent mandibular incisors and all canines and premolars was calculated with vernier calipers. Prediction tables were constructed, and they were practically identical to those of Moyers. Accordingly, either set of percentiles Moyers's or those in the present study seem to be equally appropriate to a contemporary population. However, neither method of estimation is necessary. The size in millimeters of unerupted canines and premolars at the 75th percentile can be predicted by taking half the width of the mandibular incisors and adding 11.0 for the maxillary teeth and 10.5 for the mandibular teeth..

Kaplan R. G. et al (1977)[14] the accuracy of prediction of three mixed dentition analyses was compared. Hixon and Oldfather's method was found to be the most accurate. The data were collected from dental study casts and intraoral periapical radiographs of 104 children (51 females and 53 males) selected from the longitudinal growth study conducted by the Child Study Clinic at the School of Dentistry, University of Oregon Health Sciences Center. The mixed dentition records were taken at ages ranging from 5 years 10 months to 10 years 11 months (mean, 7 years 6 months). Predicted values for the sum of the mesiodistal widths of the permanent canine, first and second premolars were calculated for the Hixon-Oldfather analysis, the Moyers analysis at the 95%, 85%, 75% and 65% probability levels and for Tanaka-Johnston's method. The results of this study indicate that the Hixon-Oldfather analysis was the most accurate of the three methods for predicting the size of the unerupted permanent canine, first and second premolars. This analysis produce a correlation coefficient that was higher and a mean difference between actual and predicted values that was significantly less than those obtained by Moyers' and Tanaka-Johnston's methods.

Ingervall et al (1978)[15] investigates with the aid of multiple regression, that which parameters of the mixed dentition were most useful for predicting the breadths of unerupted canines and premolars. They conducted a study on 77 children (38 boys and 39 girls), aged 9 years, 1 month to 10 years, 10 months (mean 10 years, 1 month). The breadth of the individual teeth in the original casts and of the canines and premolars in the roentgenograms were used as predictors of the mesiodistal breadths of t1he permanent canines and premolars. The total breadths of the upper and lower incisors, respectively, were also used as predictors. In step 1 the program used selects the predictor variable with greatest value for prediction of the dependent variable and in step 2 and subsequent steps the next most useful variable. Since the regression was linear, a multiple normal distribution was presumed for statistical test. Best results were obtained with measurement of the breadths of the teeth in roentgenograms.

Gardner R.et al (1979)[16] compared four arch length prediction equations (Nance, Johnston-Tanaka, Moyers, and Hixon-Oldfather) by examining pretreatment casts, pretreatment intraoral radiographs, and posttreatment casts of forty-one patients of mixed-dentition age. Comparison of correlation coefficients and slopes of the predicted arch length versus the actual arch lengths revealed that the Hixon-Oldfather method conformed closest to the ideal. No combination of the four methods produced a more accurate equation than the single most accurate method. Neither the sex of the patient nor the type of occlusion affected the prediction accuracy of any of the four equations.

All methods tend to overpredict the arch length size by, 1 to 3 mm with the exception of the Hixon-Oldfather equation, which underpredicted by approximately 0.5 mm. An analysis of the intra-investigator error showed a very low standard error of estimate for individual tooth measurements and for the prediction values. A variance analysis showed that most of the variation was due to arch length(85 percent), a slight amount was due to the prediction method (8 percent), and 6 percent of the variation was due to the rater. A low correlation was found between space available versus actual discrepancy and space available versus actual arch length. High correlation coefficients were found for the predicted arch lengths when compared with the actual arch lengths and the correlation coefficients for the predicted widths of only the canines and premolars compared with the actual widths were not quite as high.

Staley R.N. et al (1979)[17] investigates to determine whether, with multiple regression analysis, a more accurate method than other available methods for predicting the widths of unerupted mandibular canines and premolars of mixed-dentition patients could be developed. Regression analyses were performed on data derived from 83 Caucasian subjects (42 males and 41 females) who participated in the Iowa Growth Study. Measurements were taken on plaster casts of the mandibular incisors, canines, premolars, and first molars. Measurements of the mandibular canines, premolars, and first molars were obtained, from periapical radiographs taken with a long-cone technique. Newly developed regression equations for each sex had the highest correlation coefficients and smallest absolute errors of estimate when compared to previously published methods. The new equations and previous prediction methods were tested on a sample of 55 orthodontic patients (23 males and 32 females). The newly developed equations were also the most accurate method of prediction in the orthodontic patient sample.

Staley R. et al (1980)[18] they revised the Hixon and Oldfather method and the measurements obtained from the persons who participated in the Iowa facial growth study, are the same group of the subjects were used originally by Hixon and Oldfather to develop their prediction equation. A significantly improved prediction equation was developed. A graph was made for clinical use in the prediction of mandibular canine and premolar widths in mixed dentition patients.

Frankel H. et al (1986)[19] performed the mixed dentition analysis described by Moyers, and later validated by Tanaka on 80 American blacks to compare prediction equations between Caucasians and blacks. For the black sample, separate regression formulas were determined for the 39 males and 41 females and the combined black sample. Although sexual dimorphism of tooth size was not a consideration in the Moyers prediction charts, this research evaluated the effect of sexual dimorphism in the mixed dentition analysis. Regression equations were generated and used to determine significant differences between 2 equations for the same arch. The findings include a significant difference for the mandibular regression equation for black males when compared with (1) the Tanaka equation for Caucasians, and (2) the regression equation for black females. Maxillary regression equations were not significantly different between the Caucasian and black samples or between black males and females.

Merrified L.L. et al (1994)[20] linked clinical researches to fundamental orthodontic concepts to give the clinician a workable differential diagnosis system. The clinical research, conducted by the Charles Tweed Foundation, attempted to establish a "profile" for the Class II malocclusion correction that because of certain characteristics was destined to failure. The Cranial Facial Dental Analysis integrates this clinical research with the total space analysis to give the clinical orthodontist a useful tool for differential diagnosis.

IRWIN R.D. et al (1995)[8] evaluated the methods that have been proposed for mixed dentition analysis. They concluded that prediction of the space required in the dental arch for unerupted permanent canines and premolars has been based either on the correlation between the mesio-distal widths of these teeth and of erupted mandibular incisors, or on measurements of the unerupted teeth on radiographs. Studies comparing the different methods have shown that the method of Hixon & Oldfather (1958), as refined by Staley & Kerber (1980), was the most accurate.

Tollaro I. et al (1996)[21] investigated a sample of 60 Class II, Division 1 subjects during the mixed dentition phase. Posterior transverse interarch discrepancy (PTID) was measured as the difference between the maxillary and mandibular intermolar widths between two main groups: Class II group 1 (30 subjects) with PTID and Class II group 2 (30 subjects) without PTID. A sample of 30 Class I subjects in the mixed dentition phase was used as a control group. In Class II group 1, PTID was found to be due to a significantly narrower maxillary arch. The craniofacial skeletal features of both Class II groups and of the Class I group were assessed. The Class II group with PTID showed mandibular retrusion associated with a posteriorly displaced mandible of normal size (functional mandibular retrusion). The Class II group without PTID had mandibular retrusion due to a micrognathic mandible (anatomic mandibular retrusion). The relevance of these findings for treatment planning in Class II, Division 1 malocclusion in the mixed dentition was stressed.

Davidovitch M. et al (1997)[22] studied the effects of 6 months of continuous lip bumper therapy on patients in the mixed dentition with mild-to-moderate mandibular arch perimeter deficiency. Thirty-four patients, ages 7.9 to 13.1 years (~ = 10.2), seeking treatment in the postgraduate orthodontic clinic of the Medical College of Virginia, presented possessing 3 to 8 mm of mandibular crowding, with both mandibular primary second molars, were randomly placed in either the treatment or nontreatment group. Treated subjects underwent continuous lip bumper therapy, whereas the control subjects were monitored without undergoing any active treatment, each for 6 months. Arch dimension changes were assessed with study models. Alterations of mandibular incisor position were measured from lateral cephalometric radiographs. Mandibular left permanent first molar position changes were determined from both lateral cephalometric and tomographic radiographs, with the resolution of each imaging technique in measuring molar tooth movement also compared. It was found that significant differences in mandibular incisor inclination, molar position, arch length, and arch perimeter existed between treated and untreated subjects.

Schirmer UR et al (1997)[23] collected data from a series of 100 randomly selected study models of black patients. The sample was equally subdivided by gender and all subjects had Angle Class I molar relationships with only minor malocclusions such as minor crowding, rotations, or diastemas. Intra-examiner and inter-examiner reliability was determined at 0.2 mm. All teeth to and including the first molars were measured. These data were then utilized in regression equations for both maxillary and mandibular arches, to enable the prediction of the mesiodistal widths of the canines and two premolars. The equations and predicted values were compared with those of the Moyers' probability tables, and significant differences ($p<0.05$) were found (except for the prediction of maxillary canines and premolars in females at the 85 and 95percentile probability level). New probability tables for black subjects were formulated. It is envisaged that the proposed probability tables would be more accurate for black patients of African ancestry.

Lee-Chan S (1998)[24] conducted a study in which, 201 dental plaster casts of Asia-Pacific-American subjects, all of whom were under the age of 21 years, were used. The actual measurements were compared with the predicted values derived from the Tanaka and Johnston equations and significant differences were found. The data illustrate the limitations of the Tanaka and Johnston method when applied to a sample population of other than European descent. From this data, two linear regression equations were developed for tooth size prediction in Asian-American children.

Bishara S.E et al (1998)[3] compared two mixed dentition prediction methods that do not require the use of periapical radiographs of the unerupted permanent teeth. The two methods compared were the Tanaka/Johnston and the Boston University Prediction approaches. Records on 33 male and 22 female subjects who were participants in the Iowa Longitudinal Growth Study were used in the present study. The findings indicated that on the average the Tanaka/Johnston approach slightly overestimated the tooth size of the unerupted teeth (7 = 1.1 ± 0.9 mm). On the other hand, the Boston University approach slightly underestimated the tooth size of the unerupted teeth (7 = -0.1 ± 1.2 mm). The findings further indicated that there were statistically significant correlations between the predicted and actual tooth size. In general the r values were higher for the Tanaka/Johnston method than with the Boston University approach. Depending on the stage of dental development, i.e., which deciduous and permanent teeth are present, the Tanaka/Johnston approach can be used when the four mandibular incisors have completely erupted, whereas the Boston University approach can be used when all the deciduous canines and first molars are still present.

Nagan P, Alkire RG, Fields H Jr. (1999)[25] stated that an understanding of the dental development in primary and mixed dentitions can help in deciding when and how to intercept the malocclusion if crowding is detected. Most crowding problems with less than 4.5 millimeters can be resolved through preservation of the leeway space, regaining space or limited expansion in the late mixed dentition. In cases with 5 to 9 mm of crowding, some can be approached with expansion after thorough diagnosis and treatment planning Most of these cases will require extraction of permanent teeth to preserve facial esthetics and the integrity of the supporting soft tissue. Serial extraction or guidance of eruption is reserved for treatment of severe tooth-size/arch-size discrepancies. Space maintenance in the developing dentition can prevent unnecessary loss in arch length.

Bondarets N. et al (2000)[26] examined the lateral cephalograms of Russian patients in the following categories: control with acceptable occlusions (group 1); severe hypodontia with absence of six or more teeth (group 2); and severe hypodontia associated with hypohidrotic ectodermal dysplasia (HED) (group 3). Analysis was in a cross-sectional manner, comparing dimensions at the start of the mixed dentition phase (age 6–10) and in the permanent dentition (age 12–18). The groups were matched for age and sex. Thirty-one hard- and soft-tissue landmarks were traced, and 35 linear, 19 angular, and 7 ratioed measurements were taken and compared, using analysis of variance to compare the means of each group. A reduced anterior face height was found in groups 2 and 3 as a consequence of a reduced anterior lower face height. In group 2 in the mixed dentition, the posterior face height was also reduced. The facial profile appeared flat or concave. The subnasion point was behind the aesthetic line (EL), and in group 2 patients the naso-labial angle was obtuse when compared to nonaffected patients. In group 3 patients, the naso-labial angle became acute and lips were protuberant and everted as a consequence of the reduced vertical height. Groups 2 and 3 have the typical facial characteristics unique to hypodontia, with reduced vertical dimensions as a consequence of limited alveolar bone growth. However, group 3 patients have a unique abnormal craniofacial development.

WahabNourallah A et al (2002)[27] conducted a study with the aim to validate Tanaka and Johnston's analysis on 600 Syrian patients aged 14–22 years. Tanaka and Johnston's tables, equations, and approximations were modified in order to improve the accuracy of the prediction. The correlation coefficients found between the size of the permanent mandibular central incisors and maxillary first molars (31, 41, 16, and 26) and the maxillary and mandibular canines and premolars were high (r = .72 and .74, respectively). New, more accurate prediction tables applicable at earlier ages, and new regression equations were constructed. In addition, new easier approximations were developed to allow the prediction of the size of the unerupted maxillary canines and premolars by adding 6 mm to the half-widths of teeth 31, 41, 16, and 26. The analogous prediction of the size of the unerupted mandibular canines and premolars was obtained by adding 5.5 mm to the half-widths of same teeth, 31, 41, 16, and 26.

Tootla R. et al (2003)[28] conducted a study that compares the accuracy of space prediction for the unerupted permanent canines and premolars by (Moyers technique) and estimation by simple visual observation (SVO).Twenty clinicians with varying levels of dental experience and training blindly assessed the study models of 4 intact arches (2 maxillary and 2 mandibular) from 3 patients in the mixed dentition using both Moyers and SVO (simple visual observation) space prediction methods. Corresponding full-mouth panoramic radiographs were available for each case. Follow-up records of the eventual outcome in the permanent dentition for each case available (study models prior to any form of orthodontic intervention) served as the standard for comparison of the space predictions made. Predictions by both methods were compared with each other as well as with the eventual space situation in the permanent dentition. The differences in overall mean space prediction between the Moyers technique (excluding molar shift) and SVO ranged between 3.67 mm to 6.9 mm (lower arches) and 4.3 mm to 4.8 mm (upper arches). Generally, more crowding was estimated with the SVO method's predictions. However, the inclusion of molar shift in the Moyers analysis resulted in the prediction of more crowding in the mandible compared to SVO and eventual outcome in the permanent dentition. The range and variability in predictions were always smaller with the Moyers technique compared to SVO. Neither technique's mean space prediction more closely resembled the eventual space situation in the permanent dentition. It is concluded that although the Moyers technique demonstrated less variation and more reproducibility than SVO in its space predictions, neither of the techniques was any more accurate in predicting the final space outcome in the permanent dentition.

Buwembo W et al (2004)[29] conducted a meta-analysis to assess the applicability of Moyer's method in different ethnic groups , they included seven articles in the study by a literature search of Medline (1966–June 2003). 195 articles were reviewed and meta-analyzed. Separation of the articles into Caucasian and Asian groups gave borderline p-values of 0.05. Variation in the correlation coefficients of different populations using Moyer's method may fall either side. This implies that Moyer's method of prediction may have population variations. For one to be sure of the accuracy while using Moyer's method it may be safer to develop prediction tables for specific populations. Thus Moyer's method cannot universally be applied without question.

Kechik D. et al (2007)[30] examined in detail about the morphologic, skeletal, dental, and functional effects of functional posterior crossbite (FPXB), and the effects of maxillary expansion treatment with quad-helix appliance. The experimental group consisted of 35 FPXB patients (20 girls, 15 boys) having a mean age of 10.6 _ 1.4 years; the control group consisted of 31 normocclusive subjects (18 girls, 13 boys) with a mean age of 9.8 _ 1.6 years. Lateral, posteroanterior, and submentovertex cephalograms, transcranial temporomandibular joint radiographs, joint vibration analysis, and electromyographic recordings were obtained from every patient before and after maxillary expansion. Magnetic resonance images were taken before treatment for diagnostic purposes. These data were collected at 1 time point in the controls. Results showed that the pretreatment posteroanterior, submentovertex, and transcranial temporomandibular joint radiographs showed mandibular asymmetry relative to the cranial base and condylar malpositioning in the glenoid fossa. Joint vibration analysis findings showed different vibrations between the crossbite and noncrossbite sides, and imbalanced electromyographic findings in the experimental group. After treatment, the asymmetric morphology and position of the mandible and condyles were eliminated, and the stomatognathic system functions were normalized. It was concluded that early orthodontic treatment of FPXB creates optimum conditions for normal growth of the craniofacial skeleton and normal function of the stomatognathic system.

Akcam M.O et al (2008)[31] Conducted a study to evaluate 3-dimensional (3D) tooth crown sizes in patients with cleft lip and palate (CLP) and to compare them with those of a Class I control group. Orthodontic dental casts were used of 72 subjects with CLP (20 bilateral [BCLP], 34 unilateral left [ULCLP], 18 unilateral right [URCLP]) and 53 adolescents in the permanent dentition stage with Class I occlusion. Mesiodistal (MD), labiolingual (LL), and occlusogingival (OG) measurements were recorded by the same examiner using a digital caliper. Statistical analyses were conducted .It was concluded that Maxillary and mandibular premolar MD dimensions were larger in the CLP groups than in the control group. The smallest MD dimensions were those of the maxillary right lateral incisors in the BCLP group (*P* _0.05). The maxillary left lateral incisor MD dimensions in the ULCLP group were smaller when compared with other CLP groups (*P* _0.001). In general, MD, LL, and OG dimensions of CLP patients were smaller than those of the Class I subjects, not only in the affected maxillary dental arch, but also in the mandibular dental arch. Variations in 3D tooth dimensions were found among all CLP types. The lateral incisor in the cleft region was the smallest. Hence, 3D tooth-size evaluation should be included in the diagnostic records to determine precise treatment planning and final occlusion in CLP patients.

Durgekar SG et al (2009)[32] conducted a study to test the reliability of Moyers mixed dentition analysis in school children in Belgaum, Karnataka, India in 150 school children within the age group of 13 to 16 years old who had all permanent teeth were included. Mesiodistal dimensions of permanent mandibular incisors, maxillary and mandibular canines, and premolars were measured using a digital caliper with a resolution of 0.01 mm. The actual measurements were compared with the predicted values obtained with the Moyers prediction tables at the 35th, 50th, and 75th percentile confidence levels. Using this data, linear regression equations were formulated for tooth size prediction. The coefficient of determination [r2] was calculated to find the accuracy of the formulated prediction equations. The standard error of estimate (SEE) was calculated to determine the validity of the proposed equations. Moyers prediction tables are not an accurate method to estimate tooth dimension in our samples. The mesiodistal crown dimension in the buccal segment of the mandibular arch was larger in males (p=0.04) than in females. They concluded that the differences between predicted values from the Moyers tables and that of the present investigation are the result of racial and ethnic diversity. The accuracy of the prediction equation should be tested in a larger sample.

Cattaneo C. et al (2010)[33] was conducted a study to determine which group of permanent teeth presented the best prediction capability for the width sums of the unerupted canine and premolars in an Italian sample. A total of 150 subjects with complete permanent dentition were selected. Their dental casts were measured to 0.01 mm with a digital caliper and statistical analysis was done. The combination of the sums of the four lower incisors and the first upper molars showed the best prediction capability for the sum of permanent canines and premolars (SPCP) in the Italian sample. Moreover new regression equations were formulated including sex and arch as additional predictor variables. In 80% of the cases, estimated differences between the predicted and the actual values were smaller than 1 mm and It can be concluded that the new regression equations proposed seemed to show good accuracy.

Felicio LG. et al (2010)[34] conducted a study to evaluate the method for mixed-dentition analysis using Cone-Beam Computed Tomography for assessing the diameter of intra-osseous teeth and compare the results with those obtained by Moyers, Tanaka-Johnston, and 45-degree oblique radiographs. Measurements of mesial-distal diameters of erupted lower permanent incisors were made on plaster cast models by using a digital calliper, whereas assessment of the size of non-erupted permanent pre-molars and canines was performed by using Moyer's table and Tanaka-Johnston's prediction formula. For 45-degree oblique radiographs, both canines and pre-molars were measured by using the same instrument. For tomographs, the same dental units were gauged by means of Dolphin software resources. Statistic analysis revealed high agreement between tomographic and radiographic methods, and low agreement between tomographs and other methods being evaluated. It was concluded that Cone-Beam Computed Tomography was accurate for mixed-dentition analysis in addition to presenting some advantages over compared measurement methods ,observation and measurement of intra-osseous teeth individually with the possibility, however, to view them from different prospects and without superimposition of anatomical structures.

Philip NI et al (2010)[35] collected odontometric data from 300 male and 300 female subjects of Indian descent, who had fully erupted mandibular permanent incisors and maxillary and mandibular canines and premolars. They measured the mesiodistal crown widths with Vernier calipers. All tooth groups showed significant differences (P\0.001) between mesiodistal widths of male and female subjects. Regression equations for the maxillary arch (males, $Y = 7.15 + 0.67X$; females, $Y = 7.44 + 0.65X$) and the mandibular arch (males, $Y = 5.55 + 0.71X$; females, $Y = 6.15 + 0.67X$) were used to develop new probability tables on the Moyers pattern. Significant differences (P \0.05) were found between our predicted widths and the Moyers tables at almost all percentile levels, including the recommended 75% and 50% levels. These new prediction aids could be considered for a more precise mixed dentition space analysis in Indian children.

Berwani A.K. et al (2013)[36] conducted a study to produce simple linear equations and tables for Pakistani children. Two hundred subjects of Pakistani descent who met their criteria (ages, 13-15 years; 100 boys, 100 girls) were selected from local schools. The mesiodistal widths of all mandibular permanent incisors, canines, and premolars were measured and analyzed. The results were also compared with predicted values from the Moyers and the Tanaka and Johnston methods. Correlation and linear regression analyses were performed between the predicted and actual tooth sizes for Pakistani children and standard regression equations were developed. No significant differences were observed for measured canine and premolar antimeres and sex. Significant and high positive correlations were found between the mandibular incisors and the combined mesiodistal widths of the canines and premolarsfor the maxillary (r 5 0.65; P\0.001) and mandibular (r 5 0.59; P\0.001) segments. They concluded that the equations and charts commonly used for North American children (75th percentile) did not accurately predict for their sample. The regression equations and tables developed in this study can be used for orthodontic treatment planning for children in Pakistan.

Butt S. et al (2012)[37] During mixed dentition period, discrepancy between spaces available and required in the arch is predicted so that teeth can erupt freely with good alignment. Mixed dentition space analysis is done for this purpose in which size of unerupted canine and premolars is predicted. Accurate prediction is very important regarding correct orthodontic diagnosis and treatment planning. Prediction equation and or tables based on size of already erupted permanent teeth are the most widely used methods. Tooth size varies in different racial and ethnic groups and among genders so prediction equation and tables specific to each population for both male and female must be made. Mandibular incisors; combination of mandibular incisors and mandibular 1st molars; and mandibular incisors and maxillary 1st molars have been used worldwide. Recent studies have reported that mandibular incisors are not the best predictors and sum of mandibular incisors and maxillary 1st molars are even more accurate predictor for the estimation of size of unerupted teeth.

khanehmasjedi M. et al(2013)[38] conducted a study to determine the modified equations from Tanaka and Johnston for Iranian population. This study was an analytic and cross-sectional investigation with the randomized cluster sampling in Ahwaz. Fifty four students of 14-18 years age (32 girls, 22 boys) were selected between 320 students and plaster models of their maxillary and mandibular arches were prepared. Subjects had fully erupted teeth, class I canine and molar relationship and presented no proximal caries or fillings, morphological anomalies, missing teeth or occlusal abrasion, and bruxism. The mesiodistal crown diameters of the permanent teeth were measured with using the sharpened boley gauge (accuracy 0.01 mm). The data were analyzed by using the regression correlation analyses. The size of permanent canines and premolars were larger in maxilla than mandible and males than females. These values in Iran were different from other countries. In this study to predict the space (in mm) required for alignment of unerupted canine and premolars in Iranian children, halve the sum of mesiodistal dimension of the four mandibular incisors and add the respective constants 10.5 for upper jaw and 10 for lower jaw.

Galvão MD et al (2013)[39] conducted a systematic review in which computerized search involved articles published on PubMed and Lilacs between 1990 and September, 2011 in accordance with the method described in the Cochrane 5.1.0 handbook. The research resulted in a sample composed of 629 articles. The inclusion criteria were Articles using the Moyers analysis with a sample greater or equal to 40 patients. For this systematic review, 19 articles were selected. Based on the literature available, it was concluded that the Moyers mixed dentition analysis must be carefully used, since the majority of the articles analyzed showed that the probability of 75% was not as accurate as expected, leading to the need of adapting the probability levels depending on the study population.

Shah S et al (2013)[40] conducted a study with the aim to evaluate the accuracy of Melgaço's method in comparison with Moyers' mixed dentition analysis table in contemporary Indian population. Sixty boys and 60 girls from Gandhinagar district (age ranged from 12 to 14 years) were included. The mesiodistal crown widths of all fully erupted teeth were measured with digital vernier calipers and the odontometric values obtained were then subjected to statistical and linear regression analysis. Student's unpaired *t*-test gave statistically significant difference between the original values of teeth and the values obtained by Melgaço's prediction equation as well as Moyers' mixed dentition analysis table ($P < 0.001$). High values of correlation ($r = 0.77$) and determination coefficients ($r^2 = 0.59$) were found while considering Melgaço's method. Also, no statistically significant difference was found between the tooth sizes of males and females. It can be evaluated that Melgaço's method gives better prediction and a simplified equation $Y = 0.925X$ can be suggested for the present population.

Kaur A et al (2014)[41] conducted a study that was aimed to determine the applicability of Moyers mixed dentition arch analysis in children of Baddi, Himachal Pradesh. Dental study models of 120 children in age group of 13- 16 years, were analysed who presented with complete eruption of permanent mandibular incisors, maxillary and mandibular canines & premolars. Measurements of the mesiodistal dimensions of the mandibular and maxillary teeth were made using a digital caliper with a Vernier scale that was calibrated to the nearest 0.01mm. All tooth groups showed highly significant differences ($p<0.001$) between mesiodistal widths in male and female subjects. Significant differences ($p<0.05$) were found between actual widths and the Moyers tables at almost all percentile levels, including the recommended 75%. The differences noted might be the result of racial and ethnic diversity.

Cruz BS et al (2014)[42] In order to determine the reliability between two methodologically different method, they evaluated the systematic and random errors of the method proposed by Tanaka and Johnston, which is based on the sum of mandibular permanent incisors, and the Huckaba method, which uses radiographs. In a random sample of 28 plaster models of mandibular dental arches belonging to individuals of both genders, aged six to eleven years old, a single investigator performed the measurement of required space, according to the two methods evaluated. After 15 days, the measurements were repeated, and each of them was performed twice in sequence to calculate the repeatability and reproducibility conditions, and the systematic and random errors for each method. The random error of the method proposed by Huckaba was larger in terms of reproducibility (1.53 mm) and repeatability (0.57 mm) compared with the analysis proposed by Tanaka and Johnston (0.20 mm and 0.12 mm, respectively). The method proposed by Huckaba was proved to be inadequate in relation to reproducibility, with respect to the random error, and should be used with caution to measure the required space in the mandibular arch.

Ramesh N. et al(2014)[43] evaluates the reliability of Tanaka - Johnston and Moyer's (75th percentile) mixed dentition prediction methods in Kodava population sample, to formulate regression equations for predicting the mesiodistal widths of unerupted canines and premolars and to construct probability tables for the Kodava population. Dental models of 30 male and 30 female Kodava subjects (age range is 16 - 23 yr) were used. Teeth measured included mandibular permanent incisors, maxillary and mandibular permanent canines, first and second premolars. Digital caliper calibrated to 0.01mm was used to record mesiodistal dimensions. The actual teeth measurements were then statistically compared with the predicted values derived from the Tanaka and Johnston's equations and Moyers probability tables at the 75th percentile. Descriptive statistics including means, standard deviations were calculated for the actual and predicted tooth sizes .Tanaka and Johnston prediction equations overestimated in both the arches. Moyers 75th percentile also overestimated the actual measurements except for the maxillary arch in female subjects. The percentage of overestimation was more for Tanaka – Johnston prediction method than that of Moyers (75th percentile). Correlation and regression analysis were performed between the predicted and actual tooth size and standard regression equations were developed for the Kodava population. Probability tables were also constructed from the data obtained.

Thimmegowda UM et al (2015)[44] collected data from study models of 400 randomly selected Bangalore subjects aged 13 to 16 years with fully erupted, intact dentitions and no significant malocclusion. The mesiodistal widths of the incisors, canines and premolars of both arches were measured. This data was then utilized to predict the mesiodistal widths of canines and premolars and further compared with Moyer's table. It was found that 50% is more applicable to boys and 75% to girls. The canine premolar segment in both arches is statistically larger in men than in women ($p<0.05$). New regression equation was formulated, the accuracy of which needs to be evaluated further in a larger sample.

Hambire C.H. et al (2015)[45] carried out a study to determine the correlation between the sum of the mandibular permanent incisors and the combined mesiodistal crown diameters of the maxillary and mandibular canine and premolars in a sample of mixed Indian subjects, examine the applicability of the Tanaka and Johnston method of prediction in a mixed Indian population and develop a new prediction method for this specific population. The dental models of the dentition of 251 mixed Indian patients below the age of 21 years, who had upper and lower permanent canines and premolars erupted were selected for this study. All the measurements were made with modified Boley gauge with Vernier caliper. The differences between the predicted widths of the canine and premolars with the Tanaka and Johnston equations and the actual widths were highly statistically significant. The actual widths of the maxillary canine and premolars showed a significant difference in size from the widths predicted by the Tanaka and Johnston equation, as did the canine and premolars in the mandible. The findings suggest that the accuracy of originally derived Tanaka and Johnston mixed dentition analysis method can be increased using a newly derived regression equations based on a local mixed Indian population.

Maroli S et al (2015)[46] conducted a study to evaluate the applicability of Moyers' mixed dentition analysis to Bengali and Keralite population, to assess the percentage probability to be used for the two populations Bengali and Keralite. Record casts of 100 Bengali and Keralite (50 - Males; 50 - Females) of 12-14 years were selected, and mesiodistal width of permanent incisors, canines, premolars was measured on study models. Study models of 50 males and 50 females were prepared, and measurements were made. Paired t-test of difference between actual and predicted values for Bengali samples were least in case of the 65th percentile of the level of significance in upper arch and in lower arch it was the 50th percentile level of significance. For females, mean difference of upper arch was least at 65th percentile level and for lower arch at 50th percentile level of significance. For Keralite population, it was at 50th percentile level of significance in upper and lower arch for male and female it was at 65th percentile level in upper arch and 50th percentile level in the lower arch. The predicted value and the actual value were significantly correlated and may be used with much confidence in estimating the width of permanent canine, first premolar, and second premolar.

Mageet AO et al (2017)[47] conducted a research to determine the extent and prevalence in a representative orthodontic population in Sudan and to investigate the dimensions of TSD (tooth size discrepancy) in this population that comprised a clinically significant factor. The sample comprised 107 pretreatment study casts with fully erupted and complete permanent dentitions from first molar to first molar, which were selected randomly from records of the orthodontic patients. The mesiodistal diameters of the teeth were measured at contact points using a stainless steel digital caliper and Bolton analysis was carried out on them. A clinically and statistically significant anterior TSD (tooth size discrepancy) existed in comparison to Bolton's anterior tooth ratio. Measurements of the overall and anterior TSD (tooth size discrepancy) between malocclusion groups showed no significant differences. In terms of gender, no significant differences were observed for the overall TSD (tooth size discrepancy) data.

In Class II division 1 mean overall ratio was lower than Bolton's, and Class II division 2 mean overall ratio higher than Bolton's anterior ratio. It was concluded that Class II division 1 patients showed a tendency towards excessive maxillary tooth material and Class II division 2 patients showed a tendency towards excessive mandibular tooth material.

DISCUSSION

SPACE ANALYSIS

Proper alignment of the teeth requires harmony between the tooth sizes and the space required within the dental arch. Sometimes the space available is not similar to the space required for the alignment of the teeth. To accomplish this, a space analysis must be done. Thus it is important for the clinician to determine prior to onset of the orthodontic treatment and the space requirements necessary for favorable results.
It is important to quantify the amount of crowding within the arches because treatment varies, depending on the severity of the crowding. Space analysis using the dental casts, is required for this purpose. Such an analysis is particularly valuable in evaluating the likely degree of crowding for a child in the mixed dentition when the permanent teeth are erupting and real or transitional crowding is evident, and in that case it must include prediction of size of unerupted permanent teeth. The space analysis results must be considered in the context of the profile because reducing protrusion reduces the amount of available space. Conversely, when teeth are retroclined and then moved facially to the correct position, more space is available.

Any space management measures should be carried out only after a space discrepancy analysis is done for which the two factors to be considered are

1. Space required for proper eruption and alignment in the arch

2. Space available for the succedaneous teeth.

It can either be done by radiographic method or on study model or combination of both. For patients more than eight years of age and where the records indicated the eruption of all permanent incisors and first permanent molars, a mixed dentition analysis should be made. Several authors have recommended different analysis.

PRINCIPLES OF SPACE ANALYSIS:

Space analysis requires a comparison between the amount of space available for the alignment of teeth and the amount of space required to align them properly in dental arches. **(Figure 1)**

Since maligned or crowded teeth usually result from lack of space, this analysis is primarily of space within the arches.

This analysis can be done either

- Directly on dental casts or manually
- By computer after appropriate digitization of the arch and tooth dimension.

Whether the analysis is done manually or in the computer

The first step is to calculate the space available.

Second step is to calculate the amount of space required for alignment of teeth

First step:- Calculation of space available is accomplished by measuring arch perimeter from first molar to other, over the contact points of posterior teeth and incisal edges of anteriors.

There are two basic ways to accomplish this-

- Space available can be measured most easily by dividing the dental arch into 4 straight-line segments as shown in **(Figure 2).** Each segment is measured individually with a sharp pointed measuring instrument. (Dividers, a sharpened Boley's gauge)

- Space available can be measured by contouring.026 brass ligature wire to the line of occlusion and then straightening it out for measurement. It can also be measured by using a flexible scale.

Second step-

- To calculate the amount of space required for alignment of teeth. Measuring the M-D width of each tooth from contact point to contact point and then summing the width of the individual teeth do this**. (Figure 2)**
- If sum of the width of the permanent teeth were greater than the amount of space available there is an arch perimeter space deficiency, crowding would occur. If available space is larger than the space required gaps between some teeth would be expected.

Space analysis carried out in this way is based on three important assumptions:

(I) The anteroposterior position of the incisors is correct (i.e., the incisors are neither excessively protrusive nor retrusive),

(2) The space available will not change because of growth

(3) All the teeth are present and reasonably normal in size.

None of these assumptions can be taken for granted. All of them must be kept in mind when space analysis done.

With regard to the first assumption, it must be remembered that incisor protrusion is relatively common and that retrusion, though uncommon, does occur. There is an interaction between crowding of the teeth and protrusion or retrusion: if the incisors are positioned lingually (retruded), this accentuates any crowding; but if the incisors protrude, the potential crowding will be at least partially alleviated. Crowding and protrusion are really different aspects of the same phenomenon. If there is not enough room to properly align the teeth, the result can be crowding, protrusion, or (most likely) some combination of the two. For this reason, information about how much the incisors protrude must be available from clinical examination to evaluate the results of space analysis. This information comes from facial form analysis (or from cephalometric analysis if available).

The second assumption that space available will not change during growth is valid for most but not all children. In a child with a well-proportioned face, there is little or no tendency for the dentition to be displaced relative to the jaw during growth, but the teeth often shift anteriorly or posteriorly in a child with a jaw discrepancy. For this reasons, space analysis is less accurate and less useful for children with skeletal problems (Class II, Class III, long face, short face) than in those with good facial proportions.

Even in children with well-proportioned faces, the position of the permanent molars changes when primary molars are replaced by the premolars .If space analysis is done in the mixed dentition, it is necessary to adjust the space available measurement to reflect the shift in molar position that can be anticipated.

The third assumption can (and must) be checked by clinical and radiographic examination, looking at the teeth as a set rather than as individual units. Anomalies in tooth size have significant implications for space in the dental arches.[1]

ORTHODONTIC STUDY MODELS

Orthodontic study models are essential diagnostic records, which are accurate plaster reproductions of the teeth and their supporting soft tissues and which help to study the occlusion and dentition from all the three dimensions. Alginate impression taken for orthodontic study models should be fully extended into the buccal sulcus using suitable impression trays. In this way the teeth and supporting alveolus will readily be visible on the subsequent plaster model. Using a wax wafer the position of teeth in centric occlusion is also recorded so that the models can be hand articulated in the laboratory and Angles trimmed. Such trimming enables the static occlusal relationships of the teeth to be studied by placing the models together on the bench at a number of different angles. Steps in construction of study models: **(Figure 3-8)**

1. Impression making.
2. Taking a wax bite.
3. Disinfection of the impression.
4. Casting the impression.
5. Basing and trimming.
6. Finishing and polishing.
7. Care of the study models

Study models aid diagnosis in the following ways:

1. They enable occlusal relationships to be observed, which might not otherwise be visible. For example, where the overbite is increased, the point of contact of the lower incisor edges with the opposing arch cannot be determined clinically and yet can easily be seen on the models.
2. An accurate space analysis can be performed using models, calipers, a millimeter rule, and a piece of soft wire. The wire is used to determine arch perimeter and the calipers are used in combination with the ruler to measure the mesiodistal width of each of the teeth.
3. Models can be useful to both clinician and patient by demonstrating the effects of space closure, whether due to the developmental absence or planned extraction of teeth. Where teeth are developmentally absent the resulting space may either be closed or relocated within the arch. The effect of each treatment can be visualized be cutting the teeth off the models, moving them to the planned position and reattaching them with wax. This is known as kesling set-up.
4. Once orthodontic treatment has commenced, study models of the starting malocclusion are used to assess the progress of planned treatment changes.
5. To monitor changes in the occlusion, they are also useful as a reference to identify unwanted tooth movements.
6. On completion of treatment, study models should be obtained as a record of final result.

7. As a record required for medico-legal purposes, but the pre and post- treatment models can be used to determine the PAR (peer assessment rating) and thereby aid in audit and quality control.
8. Final models are subsequently used to monitor post treatment changes in occlusion
9. In the same way, that final models are taken at completion of treatment, in some cases models are taken but no treatment is undertaken at all. However, they can be used to monitor changes with time, either to reassure the patient that development of the occlusion is continuing satisfactorily and that no active intervention is required, or to assist the patient in the decision making processes of whether to accept or reject orthodontic treatment.

MIXED DENTITION ANALYSIS

This developmental stage begins with the eruption of the first permanent molars and continues until eruption of the premolar teeth. Determination of a definitive long term treatment plan for the patient is often not possible at this time. Not only the assessment of potential crowding or spacing within the dentition is difficult but, in some patients, particularly those with moderate class III skeletal patterns, it is difficult to estimate the long term effects of facial growth on the occlusion with any degree of certainty. However, it is possible to assist the development of the dentition by undertaking interceptive procedures. Such practices include balancing, compensating and serial extractions and are aimed at simplifying later definitive treatment in the early permanent dentition.

1. **BALANCING EXTRACTIONS**

   These are performed in order to maintain the dental centre line and can include the loss of a deciduous canine or first deciduous molar to balance the loss of the same tooth on the opposite side of the same arch. The choice of tooth for the balancing extraction will often be dictated by its prognosis and condition, but in general the deciduous canine is the balancing extraction of choice. Second deciduous molar loss is never balanced by the loss of any contralateral tooth. This is because:

   (1) The effect of second deciduous molar loss on the centre line is minimal; and

   (2) A balancing extraction of the second deciduous molar on the opposite side of the same arch can lead to rapid space loss as a result of mesial movement of the first permanent molar.

2. **COMPENSATING EXTRACTIONS**

These are carried out in opposing arches in order to maintain buccal segment relationships. They are not frequently performed.

3. **SERIAL EXTRACTIONS**

These were originally advocated by kjellgren with the stated aim of relieving crowding and allowing the development of an acceptable occlusion, without the need for extensive appliance treatment in the permanent dentition. The serial extraction regimen is:

(1) Loss of the deciduous canines around 8½ years of age, as the upper lateral incisors are erupting, in order to relieve permanent incisor crowding

(2) Loss of first deciduous molars one year later, in order to encourage the eruption of the first premolars in advance of the permanent canines

(3) Removal of the first premolars as the permanent canines are beginning to erupt, allowing the latter teeth into the line of the arch.

The classical case for serial extractions must have:

(1) A class I or mild class II or III skeletal base

(2) A class I incisor relationship; and

(3) All teeth present and in their normal developmental positions

There are a number of problems with the serial extraction regimen.

(1) In the lower arch there is no guarantee that the extraction of the first deciduous molars will encourage the first premolars to erupt before the permanent canines.

(2) In the upper arch, the premolar will erupt before the permanent canine regardless of the deciduous molar extraction.

(3) Rarely will a case meet all the correct criteria, such that following the extractions an ideal occlusion will be created without the need for appliance therapy.

(4) The child must tolerate three phases of extractions, which may necessitates subjecting the child to three general anaesthetics.

4. CORRECTION OF CROSSBITES

Generally, correction of a crossbite should take no longer than 4-6 months and is easily performed using a removable appliance.

Before embarking upon treatment it is important to determine whether there is a displacement on closing into centric occlusion. In the case of anterior crossbites, three further features should be assessed:

(1) Depth of the overbite

(2) The anteroposterior skeletal pattern

(3) The inclination of the upper and lower incisors

In case of posterior crossbites, in addition to a displacement, there should be a positive occlusal 'interlock' following upper arch expansion.

5. FUNCTIONAL APPLIANCE THERAPY

Functional appliances are used principally for the correction of moderate to severe class II division1 incisor relationships on moderate to severe class II skeletal bases. [48]

The importance of adequate space at specific times was emphasized and the critical nature of the problem, even in normal occlusions. "To treat or not treat" or "to extract" are important questions for patients between 8 and 11 years of age. The answer comes from careful study of diagnostic criteria- the patient first, together with radiographs, photographs and plaster casts. It is important to know the size of the deciduous teeth and their successors. Direct measurements in the mouth are possible and measurements of properly taken intraoral radiographs given an idea of the size of unerupted permanent teeth. Properly taken long cone technique intraoral radiographs or occlusal radiographs may be measured fairly accurately, and this exercise is to be encouraged, using fine- line dividers and a millimetre scale. Direct measurements are preferable for the most accurate appraisal. Of course, it should be remembered that rotations are difficult to measure on the two- dimensional x-ray image; distortion and continual problems. Carefully taken supplemental occlusal views can actually give even better appreciation of tooth position and size, but because of the short target film distance, some slight allowance for the magnification should be made.

Measurements on study casts are more accurate than measurements taken directly in mouth. Also, the perimeter measurement of arch length available, the mesial side of the first permanent molar, is more accurately determined on plaster cast.[49]

Indications:-

- Age group 6-12 years.
- Premature loss of primary canine.
- Rotation or blocking of lateral incisor because of lack of space.

- Ectopic eruption of permanent first molar.
- Distal terminal plane relationships.
- 1st permanent molar and permanent incisors are erupted.
- The succedaneous permanent teeth are forming.
- Size relationship between unerupted permanent teeth and primary teeth.
- There is size difference in primary canine and molars and the succedaenous teeth.
- Mesio-Distal width of primary canines and molars is greater than permanent sucessors (leeway space of nance).

Purpose of mixed dentition analysis is to evaluate the amount of space available in the arch for succeeding permanent teeth and necessary occlusal adjustments. A quantitative assessment of crowding may be obtained by mixed dentition analysis. In mixed dentition analysis mainly three factors are considered.

1. The sizes of all permanent teeth which determine – "space required' for the alignment of the teeth.
2. The arch perimeter which indicates space available for teeth alignment.

The expected changes in the arch perimeter which may occur with growth and development of occlusion

Tooth size – Arch Length Discrepancy

- Tooth size - Actual MD width measured on the model using Vernier Caliper.
- Arch length -The length of the dental arch from the distal of the last erupted tooth on one side to the distal of the last erupted tooth on the other side.

Assumptions are made in calculating a space analysis:

- All permanent teeth are developing normally & not congenitally missing
- Correlation between the size of the erupted mandibular incisors & the remaining succedaneous teeth
- Prediction tables are valid for a broad population. e.g.; most of the studies is from northwest European analysis.
- Arch dimensions remains stable throughout growth. But the intercanine width, intermolar width & arch length do change with age & eruption.
- Incisors are neither protrusive nor retrusive.

Factors to be considered in the space analysis:

The Curve of Spee- a curve of occlusion formula is used to determine the additional space required to flatten the curve of spee when required. A flat plastic square is placed on the study model, in contact with the permanent molars and mandibular incisors. The deepest point between between the plastic plate and the buccal cusps is measured with a Boley gauge. The depths of the curve on the right and left sides are added and divided by two. An additional 0.5mm is added to provide the total space required for leveling the curve of spee.

Mandibluar incisors – mandibluar incisors was mostly selected as the predictors because of higher correlation coefficient with the sum of permanent canines and premolars.

Soft tissue profile- The soft tissue profile is also an important factor to consider in the total space analysis. What actually constitutes an ideal facial balance and harmony is the most contentious aspect of the orthodontics. Because patients represent multiracial origins, a unified norm is difficult to determine.[50]

- **To predict whether there is sufficient space in the dental arch for the unerupted canines and premolars**.

  1] Measurements of the unerupted canine and premolars on radiographic images

  2] Predictions based on measurement of already erupted permanent teeth -on dental casts

  3] Combination of both

[1] Measurements of unerupted teeth on radiographs [combinations of 1&2]

A. Nance Analysis [1947]

B. Foster & Wylie [1958]

C. Hixon and Oldfather Analysis [1958]

D. Tweed's Analysis

E. Huckaba Analysis [1964]

F. Ingrevall& Lennart [1978]

G. Levern& Merrifield Analysis [1978]

[2] Predictions based on measurements of already erupted permanent teeth -on dental casts;

A. Seipel [1946]

B. Ballard & Wylie [1947]

C. Moorres [1959]

D. Tanaka and Johnston prediction value [1974]

E. Moyers analysis [1976]

Space available can be measured by dividing the dental arch into 4 straight line segments; each segment is measured individually with a sharp pointed measuring instrument. Space available can also be measured by using a flexible scale. Individual teeth dimensions can be measured using a divider or a Boley's gauge.

NANCE ANALYSIS

The Nance analysis incorporates the summation of the lower central and lateral permanent incisors (as measured from the casts) with the sum of the unerupted lower canines and premolars found on the radiographs. This yields the total space required and is compared with the total space available, as measured directly from the casts.[4]

AIM

To evaluate the amount of space available in the arch for succeeding permanent teeth and necessary occlusal adjustment

Nance's mixed dentition analysis (radiographic method), 1947

Other names

Nance- Carey's analysis

Hays and Nance analysis

ARMAMENTARIUM (Figure 12)

- Peri-apical radiograph
- Boley gauge, millimeter ruler
- Dental cast
- A piece of 0.026 inch brass ligature wire

INDICATIONS

1. Crowded or rotated permanent mandibular anterior teeth, satisfactorily placed over basal bone.
2. No marked facial deformity.
3. Mesiodistal molar relationship normal or close to normal.

4. No posterior teeth lingually or buccally placed as related to their antagonist

DETAILED PROCEDURE FOR MEASURING MESIODISTAL WIDTHS (Figure: 12-16)

- The mandibular models and the x-rays form the basis of all measurements taken.
- The dividers should be sharp-pointed for the most accurate determination of mesiodistal widths.
- Measure the mesiodistal widths of the two deciduous molars and the deciduous canine (or better, the amount of space which those teeth are occupying in the dental arch) very accurately with the dividers, and transfer the measurements to one of the ruled lines on the 3 by 5 card.
- Place an ordinary blotter beneath the card, and keep the holes pricked into the card as small as is consistent with clear visibility. As each tooth is measured, transfer the width to a line on the card and put the next tooth measurement directly in line with it so that one point of the divider enters a hole made by the previous tooth measurement.
- If a tooth is blocked out of the arch (when this occurs it is nearly always the mandibular deciduous canine), do not take the width of the tooth itself but take the space available for that tooth. For example, if the mandibular canine is excluded from the arch, then one should measure the distance from the mesial of the mandibular first deciduous molar to the distal of the mandibular permanent lateral.

- Full-mouth x-rays are used for determining the mesiodistal widths of the unerupted permanent successors.
- The accuracy of these measurements depends upon the absence of distortion in the films; therefore, x-ray technique is very important.
- The central ray of the tube should pass directly between the contact points of the teeth being x-rayed. Whether or not this has been accomplished is readily evident from inspection of the films.
- If the contact points of the teeth show no overlapping in the film, the rays have passed straight through them. If, on the other hand, the contact points have not been opened up in the x-raying, the rays have not gone straight through, and the measurements of the mesiodistal widths of these unerupted teeth are less reliable.
- The dividers are used in determining the greatest mesiodistal widths of the permanent teeth, canines and premolars, lying unerupted in their crypts.

Only cases which had good-quality pretreatment intraoral radiographs were selected. All radiographs were taken with a long-cone (16 inch) unit in order to comply with the requirements of the Nance methods of prediction. All radiographs had to be taken in such a manner as to show the greatest mesiodistal widths of the teeth in question.[16]

- When the mesiodistal widths of the deciduous and permanent teeth have been laid out on two separate lines, one may then compare the two totals.

- Two other measurements of considerable importance, should be taken from mandibular model of the mixed dentition.

- One of these is the perimeter of the arch from the mesiobuccal of one mandibular first permanent molar around to the mesiobuccal of the first molar of the opposite side. This is called simply the "outside" measurement. **(Figure 17)**

- In order to determine this, take a piece of brass wire about 0.010 inch in diameter and curve one end of it slightly, using the arch-bending pliers, so that the end curves into the embrasure and touches the mesiobuccal surface of the mandibular first permanent molar, when the main portion of the wire is lying on the middle third of the buccal surface of the second deciduous molar.

- Holding the wire in this position with the end securely against the mesiobuccal of the first molar, adapt it so that it touches the middle third of the teeth around the arch until it may be adapted into the embrasure between the mandibular second deciduous molar and first permanent molar in the same manner as the wire entered the embrasure of the opposite side, touching the mesiobuccal surface of the first permanent molar.

- When the wire has been adapted in this manner, it is cut and readapted so that the cut end exactly touches the mesiobuccal surface of the first permanent molar as it did on the opposite side. When the wire has been accurately adapted and cut off, it should be put in a coin envelope reserved for the purpose and labeled with the patient's name. It will then be available for future comparison of the length of the mixed dentition model, from molar to molar, with that of the permanent dentition model.

- Another measurement is made with the dividers and has been called the "inside" measurement.

- It is made by placing one point of the dividers at the mesiolingual of the mandibular first permanent molar of one side at the point where the lingual tissues touch the crown of the tooth.

- The dividers are then opened until the other point rests upon the gingival tissues between the mandibular central incisors at their lingual aspect. This measurement may be transferred to the card reserved for the patient, on which the mesiodistal widths of the mandibular deciduous and permanent teeth have been laid out.

RESULTS

- According to nance outside measurement will not be increased from the time of the mixed dentition to the time when all of the permanent teeth are present. Instead, there will be a definite decrease upon the succession of the permanent teeth.
- Any orthodontic procedure intended to accommodate teeth in nonrotated positions is an effort to increase this outside measurement. He found that this length cannot be permanently increased through mixed dentition treatment and that the shortening of this length observed in untreated cases is a natural and normal process and takes place in spite of treatment.

- In like manner, the inside measurement decreases. It should be understood that all comparisons are between the mandibular arch as it presents for mixed dentition treatment or observation and as it appears later when the permanent teeth have replaced the deciduous teeth. The transitional stage following mixed dentition treatment, when deciduous teeth are still present, need not concern us in a long-term analysis of any mouth.

Nance further observed that in the average patient's mandibular arch a leeway of 1.7 mm per side exists between the combined mesiodistal widths of the primary mandibular canine and first and second primary molars and the mesiodistal widths of the corresponding permanent teeth, with the primary teeth being larger. This difference in the total mesiodistal width of the corresponding three primary teeth in the maxillary arch compared with the width of the three permanent teeth that succeed them is only 0.9 mm per side.

The total predicted arch length is what is important to orthodontists and pedodontists, In as much as that value aids in the decision as to whether or not to extract teeth. The predicted total arch length takes into account the clinician's ability to measure crowding or spacing in the arch, and thus it is a better indicator than merely the predicted widths of the canines and premolars.

ADVANTAGES

- It can be performed with reliability

  It can be seen both in radiograph and on the casts, usually a primary molar tooth.

  The following formula was used to correct the radiograph errors

$X1/X2 = Y1/Y2$ or, $Y1 = X1 \times Y2/X2$

Where, X1 = true width of premolars.

X2 = apparent width of premolars.

Y1 = true width of unerupted premolar.

Y2 = apparent width of unerupted premolar.

Accuracy is fair to good, depending on the quality of the radiographic and their position in the arch. This technique can be used in maxillary and mandibular arches for all ethnic groups.

- It results in minimal errors
- It allows analysis of both arches

LIMITATION

- Complete mouth radiograph is needed
- It is time consuming
- Radiographic errors

Nance concluded, as a result of comprehensive studies, that the length of the dental arch from the mesial surface of one mandibular first permanent molar to the mesial surface of the corresponding tooth on the opposite side is always shortened during the transition from the mixed to the permanent dentition.[4]

Nance demonstrated that deficiencies of arch length could be overcome temporarily through treatment, but all too often alterations of tooth position in the post retention period brought about a return to arch dimensions equal to or less than those presenting in the original condition.[7]

Robert B. Gardner (1979) conducted a study to compare the accuracy of some of the more popular prediction methods and to determine whether a combination of methods can be used to improve upon their accuracy. The methods in question include those of Nance,' Johnston and Tanaka," Hixon and Oldfather, and Moyers. A combination of the Nance and Hixon-Oldfather methods produced the best correlation coefficients and standard errors of the estimate.[16]

Mandibular arch is used as a reference point in most prediction analyses for, as Nance' has indicated, successful mixed-dentition predictions center on analysis of the lower arch. [16]

Nance describes his method in some detail and presents clinical evidence as to why measurements taken at this relatively early age may be validly used to estimate the child's prospects for having an evenly aligned mandibular dental arch, to determine indications for present and future therapy, and to establish the necessity for the extraction of permanent teeth in the permanent dentition.[9]

The ease and accuracy with which this sort of case analysis is accomplished is greatly affected by the quality of the x-rays available for the orthodontist's use. The accuracy with which the mesiodistal widths of unerupted teeth may be determined depends in large part upon the technique with which the films were taken, but even when these variables are reduced to a minimum, teeth may be rotated in their crypts so that a true measurement of mesiodistal width cannot be determined from intraoral or extraoral films eyen when they are beyond reproach.[9]

Foster and Wylie' compared the radiograph-measurement method of Nance" with the regression equation method of Ballard and Wylie.' In a study of nineteen subjects, the radiograph-measurement method more accurately predicted the widths of the unerupted teeth than did the regression equation method. The mean absolute errors were 1.1 mm. for the radiograph method and 1.8 mm for the regression equation method. The radiograph method always overpredicted the size of teeth due to radiograph magnification.[17]

Ballard and Wylie provided a method of computing the total mesiodistal width of the unerupted mandibular canine and premolars. This procedure was devised to be used in conjunction with Nance's method of mixed dentition case analysis, in which the measurements of these three teeth, the canine and premolars, are taken from intraoral radiographs. A graph was formulated from which the mesiodistal width of the mandibular incisors had been determined.[12]

Currently the Nance arch-length analysis is seldom used, partly because the involved procedures for this analysis require a complete set of periapical radiographs. The clinical reliability of other analyses that do not use radiographs is sufficient for determining major arch-length inadequacies

FOSTER AND WYLIE ANALYSIS (1958)

- This method is recommended by HERBERT R. FOSTER AND WENDELL L. WYLIE in 1958. Shortly after the publication of Nance's article, they began a serial study of certain clinical procedures which might be profitably compared with one another and which suggested themselves in the light of Nance's findings. They Examined 72 children at 18 month intervals over a period of 10yrs.
- They estimated the size of unerupted permanent canines & premolars by 2 methods:

  1] Ballard & Wylie Method **(figure 18)**

  2] By measuring the teeth on radiographs taken using long cone technique.
- Compared these estimates with the actual sizes of the teeth after they had erupted.

AIM

(1) To evaluate the characteristics of the permanent dentition resulting from the premature removal of mandibular deciduous canines.

(2) The reliability of predicting eventual arch length from measurements made during the mixed dentition.

(3) Estimates of the mesiodistal width of unerupted canines and premolars based upon the widths of mandibular incisors, as compared with the measurement of these widths from intraoral films, and

(4) The positional changes, if any, of incisors and molars over such a span of years.

ARMAMENTARIUM

- Fine –pointed dividers
- Record card
- Plaster models
- Complete intraoral films
- Cephalometric films

PROCEDURE

- A study including 72 children in mixed dentition, with 34 at the end of study.
- In each instance complete intraoral films, cephalometric films and plaster models were obtained.
- When these records were complete, mandibular deciduous canines were removed in several children.
- In 23 cases this was done because of crowding in mandibular anterior segments, in 6 cases this was done because one deciduous canine had been lost, they sought to restore symmetry. One remaining case offered no justification for extraction.
- Average age at which deciduous canines were removed was 8 years 2 months and the average age at the time of terminal models was 12 years 8 months.
- Group A- deciduous canines were removed but no appliance was placed

  Group B- deciduous canines were removed, lingual arches were placed

  Group C-deciduous canines were removed, lingual arches were placed and permanent teeth extracted.

PREDICTION OF ARCH LENGTH

For each subject in the study, the "space available" for succedaneous teeth was determined as follows:

The mesiodistal width of each non-rotated tooth was determined by the use of fine-pointed dividers and transferred as a tiny pinhole in the record card.

↓

These were arranged in the straight line and to them were added measurements of any spaces, plus measurements of the "space occupied" by rotated teeth.

↓

It was readily seen that the total space so picked out on a line of the record card constitutes the amount of space available for succedaneous teeth, provided that their assumptions were accurate.

Their working hypothesis assumed that they are accurate but they remember that actually this distances shortens. Because they accept the arbitrary figure of Nance (1.7mm on each side) and when they determine "space available" and they deduct 3.4mm from the value obtained by the procedure described above.

Mixed dentition models permit accurate measurement of mandibular incisors.

In this study two separate methods were used for each subject for the sake of comparison:

1. Direct measurement of intraoral films
2. Predictions from Ballard –Wylie chart on models **(Figure 18)**

Any difference between "space available" and "space required" was termed was termed either "leeway" or "discrepancy" depending upon which of the two measurements was larger.

The accuracy of the measurements from mixed dentition x-rays and of the predicted value was checked by taking divider measurements from models of the same children after eruption of all the permanent teeth.

RESULTS

1. The ten subjects of Group A (who wore no lingual arches) showed an average reduction of arch length of 2.9 mm
2. Six showed a reduction less than Nance's 3.4 mm, the least being 0.9 mm.
3. The remaining four exceeded 3.4 m., with a maximum reduction of 5.2 mm. Because of the presence of lingual arches in the other two groups (and extraction of first premolars in Group C), only Group A was studied in this connection. The average age of the ten subjects in Group A was 12 years 8 months when terminal measurements were taken. **Schaeffer's** work suggests that further shortening could take place.

FACTORS AFFECTING ACCURCY OF PREDICTION

Measuring the width of a tooth on a model or on a roentgenogram may introduce an error of 0.1 mm. at each point of the dividers, for the human eye at normal viewing distance can distinguish no closer than 0.1 mm., according to determinations by Philleo"

A check on the relative accuracy of different methods of prediction based measurements, in order to be complete, should not fail to consider the degree of error introduced by measurement itself without regard to the original material being measured.

Consequently, a test was devised which utilized an easier medium than plaster models or x-ray films, namely, a metal millimeter rule in which the calibrations were engraved into the metal and filled with black enamel for contrast. To simulate the clinical situation, each man cooperating in the study was asked to sharp-pointed dividers to prick out on the line of a card a total distance of 70 mm. in the following fashion:

He would first set his dividers at 9 mm. on the metal scale

↓

Transfer the measurement to the card;

↓

Then he would set the dividers at 8, 7, 6, and 5 mm respectively, and repeat the process.

↓

This obliged him to reset the dividers after each measurement and the total distance of 70 mm. approximates the distance ordinarily encountered clinically.

↓

Accuracy of the test was appraised by measuring the distance between the first and last pinholes with the same metal scale.

One might expect that small errors introduced by the human factor would tend to cancel out, that is, errors on the small side would occur as frequently as errors of magnification. On the contrary, of the twenty tests conducted by six different persons, only two were under a total of 70 mm. one was exactly correct and the remainders were over the correct figure. The median result of twenty measurements was 70.5 mm, with a range of 69.7 to70.9 mm. This suggests that under ideal conditions the technique of transferring measurements to a line on card tends to error slightly in the direction of magnification.

CONCLUSION

1. Premature removal of primary canines has no adverse effect upon ultimate inter-canine width.

2. When premature removal of primary canines was indicated, placing a lingual arch had dubious value in this series of patients, whether it was intended to prevent lingual positioning of incisors or to prevent forward positioning of molars. Lingual arches are certainly useful where second primary molars are lost or where their loss is imminent.

3. Arch length shortens in the transition from the mixed to the permanent dentition, and the basis for this shortening differs in different persons. In most instances the shortening can be attributed more to a lingual shifting of incisors upon the symphysis rather than to a forward shift of molars.

4. Prediction of arch length deficiency in the permanent dentition, based upon measurements made during the mixed dentition, is sufficiently inaccurate that caution should be exercised in applying such predictions clinically. While mesiodistal widths of unerupted cuspids and premolars may be predicted from measurements of incisors with more accuracy than one can measure these widths in poor intraoral films, films taken by a meticulous technique can outperform the mathematical formulas. Whether films or formulas are used, however, appreciable errors in prediction can occur.

Lloyd (1956) recommends the use of the lingual arch when mandibular second deciduous molars are removed for strategic purposes. In other situations he seems to share present view that the lingual arch may often be omitted with safety in serial extraction procedures.[51]

Barrow (1952) a chart by barrow based on serial study of fifty one children with normal occlusion, shows no net change in inter-canine measurement between 8 years 2 months and 12 years 8 months.[52]

Lewis (1936) shows an increase of inter-canine measurement 1.8mm between 8 years 2 months and 12 years of age.[53]

These data suggest, when compared with present study that the premature removal of mandibular deciduous canines does not adversely affect the final mandibular intercanine width.

HIXON AND OLDFATHER, 1958

HISTORICAL REVIEW:
There has been an increased tendency in recent years to initiate orthodontic treatment during the early mixed dentition period. The trend toward earlier treatment reflects better comprehension of malocclusions and their diagnosis. In terms of treatment, Kloehn's revival of extra-oral anchorage and Kjelgren's introduction of serial extraction exemplify better understanding of strengths and limitations of current appliance therapy.

Some of the concepts underlying these therapies are:

1. Relative stability of arch width in the untreated case after the eruption of the permanent incisors
2. Slight decrease in mandibular arch length anterior to the permanent molars,
3. Inability of appliance therapy to measurably influence more than the teeth and their immediate supporting tissues
4. Undesirable effects from extensive use of mandibular anchorage.

As pointed out by Nance, diagnosis during the mixed dentition hinges to a large extent on analysis of the lower arch.

From this viewpoint, diagnostic variables to be considered are:

1. Crowding or spacing present in the mandibular arch in the mixed dentition
2. Difference between the size of unerupted cuspids and bicuspids and space in the mandibular arch available for them
3. Inclination of the incisors
4. Expected slight increase in arch width
5. Expected slight decrease in arch length anterior to the permanent molars.

From the five considerations above, first two show greatest variability and as a result, receive the most attention in diagnosis and treatment planning.

Nance, Ballard and Wylie, Carey and Griewe have previously given consideration to the problem of predicting the size of the mandibular cuspids and bicuspids before their eruption and have developed useful techniques for this purpose.

Hixon and Oldfather add the maximum mesiodistal diameters of the permanent mandibular central and lateral incisors with those of the unerupted premolars measured on the intraoral film. The summation is called the "measured value," which is used to determine the "estimated value" from prediction charts. The prediction charts compensate for magnification inherent in radiography and are valid only for measurements taken from radiographs from a long-cone (16inch) x-ray unit. The method is claimed to be accurate to within 0.6 mm. for 68 percent of the cases, 1.1 mm. for 95 percent of the cases, and 1.7 mm. for 99 percent of the cases used both radiographs and the sizes of erupted teeth.

This combines the best features of both techniques in an effort to improve predictability and yet sacrifices time saving features. The quality of intraoral films should be the determining factor in the selection of the technique over the other.

AIM:

- The primary objective of this investigation was to determine if a more efficient procedure could be found that is error in prediction could be reduced further as compared to previous studies.
- To study relationship between size of permanent cuspids and bicuspids and size of their deciduous predecessors.

ARMAMENTARIUM:

1. X –ray films
2. Hydrocal casts
3. Finely pointed Boley gauge

REQUIREMENTS:

1. A cast of the lower arch with deciduous canine and molars present, and free from proximal carious lesions.
2. Periapical x-ray film of the same side as above, taken the same date as the impression for the cast, with deciduous canine and molars present and erupted with permanent canine and premolars present but unerupted.
3. A later cast with permanent canine and premolars and incisors erupted; with no proximal carious lesions or restorations on the side measured previously.

PROCEDURE:

- A sample of forty one children, fifteen males and twenty six females, from the Facial Growth Study at the State University of Iowa met the above requirements.
- All were American-born and of predominantly northwest European ancestry.
- The teeth were measured on hydrocal casts obtained from alginate impressions.
- The intraoral x- ray films used were taken by a technician using a conventional dental x- ray machine fitted with a cone giving a 16-inch skin-target distance.
- The cast measurements of the mesial-distal diameter of the deciduous teeth and the x- ray measurements of deciduous canine and molars and permanent canine and premolars were made within one year of shedding of deciduous canine and molars.

- The age range of these measurements was from 7 years, 6 months to 11 years.
- The tooth measurements of the permanent teeth of the same individuals were obtained from casts taken 12 and 15 years of age.
- For all teeth the maximum mesial-distal diameters of the crowns of the individual teeth were measured at right angles to the long axis of tooth. A finely pointed, Boley gauge was used throughout. Where teeth were rotated before eruption, maximum crown diameter on the films measured at right angles to the long axis was considered as the width of these teeth.
- Two independent measures were recorded for each tooth. If the two measures agreed within 0.1 mm, the average of the two was used. If disagreement exceeded 0.1 mm, two more independent measures were taken and four averaged.
- Product –moment correlation coefficients of r=0.97 and r=0.99 indicate the high reliability of the two original cast and film measurements.
- Associations for the combined widths of permanent canine and premolars and each of twelve predictive combinations were obtained by preparing scattergrams and computing pearson product-moment correlation co-efficients (r). The obtained values were given in table 1.

Combined widths of 3, 4, and 5 correlated with:	*r*
c, d, e cast	.56
1, 2, 2, 1 cast	.69
3, 5 x-ray film	.78
4, 5 x-ray film	.80
3, 4 x-ray film	.82
3, 4, 5 x-ray film	.82
1, 2, 2, 1 cast plus c, d, e cast ..	.75
3, 4 x-ray film plus 1, 2, 2, 1 cast .	.84
3, 4, 5 x-ray film plus 1, 2, 2, 1 cast plus c, d, e cast	.85
4, 5 x-ray film plus 1, 2, 2, 1 cast .	.88
4, 5 x-ray film plus 1, 2 cast ...	.88*
4, 5 x-ray film plus 1, 2 cast ...	.87**
4, 5 x-ray film plus 1, 2 cast ...	.82***

- One additional approach , an attempt to correct for enlargement of permanent canine and premolars on the film by the ratio $\frac{\text{cast c, d, e}}{\text{x- ray c, d, e}}$

gave such wide dispersion on the scattergram that the correlation coefficient was not computed.

RESULTS:

- Weakest correlation coefficient was that between size of deciduous posterior that is canine and molars and permanent canine and premolars was r=0.56.
- The correlation coefficient between the sum of the widths of mandibular permanent incisors and that of mandibular permanent canines and premolars, measured on the casts, was similar to that reported by other authors (0.69).[9]
- The strongest correlation (0.88) was between, on the one hand, the sum of the widths of the central and lateral incisors in one quadrant, measured on the casts, added to the sum of the widths of the two premolars in the same quadrant, measured on radiographs, and, on the other, the sum of the widths of the canines and premolars after their eruption.
- From these results the authors devised a table for prediction of the mesio-distal widths of unerupted canines and premolars, which is shown in Table 2.[8]

Sum of mesio-distal widths of central and lateral incisors in a quadrant (measured on dental casts) plus sum of mesio-distal widths of first and second premolars in the same quadrant (measured on radiograph) (mm)	Predicted sum of mesio-distal widths of unerupted canine and premolars in the quadrant (mm)
23	18.4
24	19.0
25	19.7
26	20.3
27	21.0
28	21.6
29	22.3
30	22.9

Hixon Oldfather's probability table

- The width of incisors plus the x-ray measure of permanent premolars gave a sufficiently strong relationship to be clinically useful in predicting size of permanent canine and premolars before their eruption. Since this relationship does not involve the size of deciduous canine and molars, the restriction in sample selection with reference to restorations in the deciduous teeth could be removed. By removing this restriction an additional thirty-five subjects became available for study. The larger sample (n=76) provided a better basis for generalizing in terms of clinical use.

- The coefficient of correlation from the seventy six cases, utilizing the best film of permanent premolars available before their eruption, was r=0.87. This figure is included in table 1. In table 2, the results have been expanded for prediction purposes in clinical situations.
- The standard error of estimate for this relationship is 0.57 mm, which means the size of permanent canine and premolars can be predicted before their eruption within 0.57mm for two-thirds of the cases, and the error of prediction will not exceed 1.1mm on more than one child in twenty. The error of prediction will be as great as 1.7mm one time in 100.
- The index of forecasting efficiency is 50 per cent. This represents an improvement of more than 25 percent over methods previously suggested.
- For the sample under study the maximum error of prediction from the proposed technique was 1.2mm. Corresponding maximum errors were 2.8mm with Carey chart, 2.3mm with the Ballard and Wylie chart and 3.9 mm from x- ray measurements of permanent canines and premolars.[54]
- In mixed dentition analysis, the estimated size of permanent canine and premolars can then be compared with the space available for their eruption. this space available can be obtained by measuring from the mesial surface of the mandibular permanent molars to the distal of the lateral incisors with a Boley gauge on which the measuring blades have been ground to a fine edge.
- For alignment of teeth, compensation must then be made for incisor crowding or spacing, improper incisor inclination, plus incisal rotations. In ascertaning space for alignment, the potential mesial shift of the molars should also be considered.

- Table 3 presents singly, and in combination, the difference in tooth size found between deciduous canine and molars and their permanent succesors.

Tooth width	Mean	S.D.	Range
3-c	+1.01mm	0.39mm	+0.2 to +2.0mm
4-d	-0.60mm	0.48mm	+0.4 to -1.6mm
5-e	-2.55mm	0.42mm	-1.7 to -3.3mm
3,4,5-c,d,e	-2.13mm	1.05mm	-0.1 to -4.4mm

- On the average, the combined width of the three permanent teeth was 2.1mm smaller than that of the three deciduous teeth.
- Oldfather's method was modified by Stahle (1959) by including the sizes of the mandibular permanent incisor to predict mesiodistal width of canine and premolars.[37]
- Staley, R. N. and P. E. Kerber (1980) revised Hixon and Old Father and developed prediction equation and made a graph for the estimation of mesiodistal width of unerupted caine and premolars.[18]
- Several researchers predicted mesiodistal width of unerupted canine and premolars in Caucasian population by a combination of measurements of teeth from dental radiograph and regression analysis done on dental casts and they found it to be more accurate in their respective population.[17]

- The accuracy of prediction of three mixed dentition analysis was compared. That is Hixon and Oldfather, Moyer's and Tanaka-Johnston methods. Hixon and oldfather's method was found to be the most accurate.[14]
- While comparing the accuracy of some of the more popular prediction methods and to determine whether a combination of methods can be used to improve upon their accuracy. The methods in question include those of Nance,' Johnston and Tanaka," Hixon and Oldfather, and Moyers .All methods tend to overpredict the arch length by, 1 to 3 mm with exception of the Hixon-Oldfather equation, which underpredicted by approximately 0.5 mm.
- A combination of the Nance and Hixon-Oldfather methods produced the best correlation coefficients and standard errors of the estimate.[16]

TWEED'S ANALYSIS

This method is recommended by CHARLES H. TWEED in 1963. It is facial oriented analysis, incorporating the relations of the incisor teeth to the basal bone. This analysis is described as Tweed method.

Historically tooth size/jaw size discrepancies diagnosed in the mixed dentition period are evaluated by dental oriented analyses; these analyses will be referred to as conventional methods. Their aim was to evaluate, as accurately as possible, future crowding in the permanent dentition using a prediction of the mesiodistal width of the permanent mandibular canines and premolars. The value obtained is added to the already known measurement of the permanent mandibular incisors. This represents space required. The space required is subtracted from the arch circumference of space available. If the result is significantly negative, future crowding can be predicted.

But tweed studying the relationship between the mandibular incisors and mandibular plane, found that if the teeth are not in a stable relationship with the basal bone after treatment, the result may relapse. In view of this, the dental-oriented mixed dentition analysis alone is not adequate.

According to Tweed, an assessment of the relations between axial inclination of the mandibular incisors and the basal bone was made on tracing of the lateral cephalogram.

- The Tweed diagnostic facial triangle was concerned as a basis for diagnosis and treatment planning. It consists of

  FMA – Frankfort mandibular plane angle
  IMPA – Incisor mandibular plane angle
  FMIA – Frankfort mandibular incisor angle
  Tweed Estd. 25^0 as norm for FMA
  90^0 for IMPA
  65^0 for FMIA

  The value for space required and space available was assessed according to conventional method. The Tweed foundation research established the following relationships. **(Figure 19)**

- When (FMA) is between 21^0 - 29^0, (FMIA) should be 68^0.
- When (FMA) is 30^0 or greater , (FMIA) should be 65^0
- When (FMA) is 20^0 or less , (IMPA) should not exceed 92^0

If the cephalometric tracing did not correspond to the above objectives, an objective line was traced to form the required FMIA. Then the distension between this and the line that passed through the actual axial inclination of mandibular incisors was measured on the occlusal plane. The figure is multiplied by 2 to include right and left sides. The total is the cephalometric correction which is added to the difference got by conventional method to give the total discrepancy.

ARMAMENTARUM:

- Models
- Photographs
- Lateral cephalometric headplate
- Lateral jaw roentgenograms
- Intraoral roentgenograms

PROCEDURE:

Examine to determine the presence or absence of a deviate swallow.

↓

Secure models, photographs, a lateral cephalometric headplate, and lateral jaw and intraoral roentgenograms.

↓

Measurement of unerupted permanent teeth and recorded to determine whether or not a tooth-basal bone discrepancy exists.

↓

The diagnostic facial triangle must be drawn on the headplate to determine the amount of headplate correction.
(It is necessary to position the denture correctly in its relation to basal bones.)

↓

Presuming the case is of a discrepancy nature, a serial extraction program is begun at the age of approximately 8 years.

The sequence is as follows:

1. All four first deciduous molars are removed at the age of approximately 8 years.
2. About 4 to 10 months following extraction of the first deciduous molars the first premolars will have erupted to gingival level.
3. At this time all four erupting first premolars, along with all four deciduous canines, are removed. This must be done at least 4 to 6 months prior to eruption of the canines, which usually migrate distally and erupt into good positions.

The irregularities of the mandibular incisors, if not too severe, are self corrective.

In addition, functional denture mechanics tip these teeth lingually to inclinations in keeping with the forces to which they are subjected during normal use. There are angular changes that have occurred in the diagnostic facial triangle during the serial extraction period prior to any kind of mechanical orthodontic treatment.

In each instance the removal of all four deciduous canines and all four erupting first premolars is followed by a lingual tipping of the mandibular incisors as a result of functional denture mechanics.

Mandibular incisor inclinations that approach, much less exceed, 90 degrees when related to the mandibular plane. This self-action, translated in terms of treatment time, saves from 7 to 9 months of treatment and assures one of the correct positions and inclinations of the mandibular incisors.

CLASSIFICATION OF FACIAL GROWTH TRENDS

Growth trends may be classified into Type A, Type B, and Type C and their subdivisions.

Type A

- Growth trend of both maxilla and mandible is forward and downward, with both upper and lower face advancing in unison.
- Angle ANB remaining unchanged, the prognosis is good
- Growth processes will be advantageous for both patient and orthodontist.
- No treatment is indicated during the serial extraction period, provided that the ANB angle does not exceed 4.5 degrees.
- Treatment should not be started prior to the full eruption of all four permanent canines, at which time full appliance therapy should be instituted with headgear worn 14 hours each day.
- The prognosis is good. Facial esthetics will be very satisfactory
- Treatment time should be 15 to 18 months.

TYPE A SUBDIVISION

- If the ANB angle exceeds 4.5 degrees, the magnitude of maxillary tooth movements will be greater than in the previous case.
- Facial esthetics should be good.
- Controlled headgear treatment should be started immediately following removal of the first premolars.
- Upon complete eruption of all permanent canines, full appliance therapy should be started.
- Headgear should be worn 14 hours per day.
- Treatment time will be from 18 to 21 months.
- About 25 per cent of patients in this study have Type A growth trends.

TYPE B SUBDIVISION

- If the ANB angle is large and increasing in size during the observation period, the growth trend is most undesirable, and it cannot be expected that the mandible will be advanced as a result of treatment.
- "A" point must be moved posteriorly to reduce the size of the ANB angle.
- Such a case demands extraction of teeth, and the patient will require prolonged treatment.

- Controlled headgear treatment should be started as soon as the maxillary first premolars have been extracted under serial extraction and continued for 15 to 18 months, or until full eruption of the permanent canines, at which time full appliance therapy should be instituted.
- Total treatment time will be from 24 to 32 months. The headgear must be worn 20 hours per day.
- The magnitude of maxillary tooth movements will be enormous.
- The prognosis for dramatic facial change is not good.
- Rarely is one able to attain an FMIA of 65 degrees in these cases.
- Only 15 percent of cases in this study fall into this category.

TYPE B

- In those cases in which patients present ANB angles of less than 4 degrees, favorable facial changes and good occlusions may be expected, 'but the orthodontist must work to the best of his ability.
- It is advantageous to begin early controlled headgear treatment immediately following removal of all four erupting first premolars and all four deciduous canines.
- Upon complete eruption of all four permanent canines, full appliance therapy should be instituted.
- The headgear should be worn 14 hours per day. Treatment time will be from 18 to 21months.

TYPE C

- Growth is equally forward and downward and that the lower face is growing forward more rapidly than the upper face, with a decrease in the size of the ANB angle.
- Growth processes are favorable to both the patient and the orthodontist.
- Treatment of the case will not be difficult or lengthy, and the magnitude of maxillary tooth movements will be much less than in the previous cases.
- The prognosis is excellent and facial esthetics should be excellent.

- No treatment is indicated until the full eruption of all permanent canines.

TYPE C SUBDIVISION

- Growth is more forward than downward and that the lower face is growing forward more rapidly than the upper face, with a decrease in the size of the ANB angle.
- Growth processes are again being very kind to both patient and orthodontist.
- Treatment time should be in the neighborhood of 10 to l5 months.
- The magnitude of tooth movements will not be as great as in Type A and B growth trend cases, and one should reasonably expect lovely facial balance and stable dentures.
- In these cases, if the ANB angle is less than 4.5 degrees, treatment should not be started until the full eruption of canines, second premolars, and mandibular second permanent molars has taken place.
- Treatment time should be in the neighborhood of 10 to 15 months.
- Fortunately, 60 per cent of patients in this study are blessed with Type C growth trends.

LIMITATIONS

He was unable to correlate the type of growth trend with the size of the Frankfort-mandibular plane angle.[13]

HUCKABA ANALYSIS

- This analysis is recommended by GEORGE W. HUCKABA in 1964. This analysis makes use of a radiograph and study cast to determine the width of unerupted teeth

PURPOSE/NEED FOR ANALYSIS

- For determining some reliable means of arch size analysis and tooth size prediction.
- Such procedure should be carried out in the average dental office with the usual equipment to be found there.
- Direct intraoral measurement of the dental arches may not offer a reliable basis of judgment of arch space
- Direct measurements of the images of unerupted permanent teeth on the x-ray film are misleading because of the magnification factor.

ARMAMENTARIUM

- Periapical radiograph
- Boley gauge,
- millimeter ruler
- Dental cast

PRINCIPLE

- With any type of radiograph, it is necessary to compensate for enlargement of radiographic image .This can be done by measuring an object that can be seen both in the radiograph and on the cast, such as primary molar tooth. It is possible to determine the measurements of un- erupted teeth by studying the teeth that have already erupted in a radiograph and on a cast.

ARCH SIZE ANALYSIS

A patient in the early mixed dentition stage who presents for examination should be evaluated to determine just how many millimeters of space he will have in his dental arches to accommodate the remaining permanent teeth when they finally erupt.

It is a well established principle that there is no physiologic provision for interstitial bone growth. This means that there can be no increase in the amount of bone between the roots of adjacent teeth.

Lateral width growth anterior to the area of the first permanent molar teeth is virtually complete before age eight years. Thus we may consider that the total amount of the dental arch space available for the eruption of the remaining permanent teeth will not be increased by growth after this time.

PROCEDURE

- Measure the dental arch circumference from mesial of lower first permanent molar on one side around the arch to mesial of first permanent molar on the opposite side we will have determined the maximum arch space a patient can anticipate in the absence of orthodontic intervention.
- This arch circumference may be determined by a procedure known as the wire measurement which is carried out in the following manner:

  A length of the soft- temper wire, such as 0.25 inch diameter brass orthodontic separating wire, is adapted to lie over the proximal contact areas of the teeth present in the lower arch. In cases in which the teeth are badly crowded or overlapped, the mean alignment is used. If the teeth are upright over the bony base and in favorable axial position, the ends of the wire are cut off exactly at the mesial surfaces of the lower first permanent molar. Cases will be observed in which the incisor teeth are tipped to the lingual, indicating that they must be placed in a more upright position by labial tipping at a later time. The wire measurement in such cases is made by extending the anterior segment of the wire to the labial of the incisors to the extent of labial tooth movement anticipated. Conversely, if the teeth are tipped to the labial, then the measuring wire must be positioned to the lingual in the incisor area to allow for later lingual tipping corrections in the incisor area to allow for lateral tipping corrections. After these allowances have been made the wire is cut off at the level of the mesial surfaces of the first permanent molars. This wire, which represents the patient's total arch circumference, is straightened with the fingers and measurements with a Boley gauge, and the length is recorded.[2]

TOOTH SIZE PREDICTION

- He noted that human teeth tend to show a close correlation in proportionate size. If the central and lateral incisors show a smaller than average size, then the sizes of the canines and premolars similarly can be expected to be smaller than average.[16]
- Most of the studies have found the sum of four mandibular incisors as the best predictor for estimating the mesiodistal width of unerupted permanent canine and premolars.[55]

- This has permitted investigators to compile a prediction chart for the combined mesiodistal width of the upper or lower permanent cuspid and premolar teeth when the combined widths of the lower incisor teeth are known.
- The charts reproduced here in tables were compiled in the department of orthodontics at the University of Michigan School of dentistry.
- Measure the width of each of the four mandibular incisor teeth with a modified Boley gauge or by the use of fine- pointed dividers. A Boley gauge may be altered for the intraoral use by cutting away the calliper jaws and tapering the parallel beaks to fine points.
- The sum of these four measurements is the amount of incisor tooth material which must be accommodated in the absence of overlapping. This total incisor width is subtracted from the arch circumference which was obtained previously. The remainder is the amount of arch space available for the permanent cuspid and premolar teeth on the right and left sides of the lower dental arch. This figure is divided by two to obtain the amount of arch space currently available for the eruption of a cuspid and two premolar teeth on each side of the arch.
- Now consult the probability chart for predicting the sum of the widths of $\overline{345}$ from $\overline{21|}12$. Across the top of the chart is a series of figures representing combined width of the lower incisors designed as Ɛ $\overline{21|\ 12}$. Locate the measurement which corresponds most closely to the sum of the incisor teeth of case in question. Read vertically down the column until the figure nearest the arch space for cuspid and bicuspid teeth was found. Then read horizontally to the column on the extreme left, which will be a percentage which represents the probability that the

patient in question will have adequate space for his remaining permanent teeth, assuming that no drift of the first permanent molars was permitted.

INTERPRETATION OF FINDINGS

The routine just outlined offers the dentist a simple and valuable diagnostic tool which will enable him to place a given patient in one of three groups that is:

1. The dental arches are of sufficient size to accommodate all the teeth, and amount of excess space is indicated.
2. The dental arches are inadequate to accommodate all the permanent teeth, and the approximate extent of the deficiency is indicated.
3. The patient falls within the probability area of the chart in which case there is some question whether there will be space for the eruption of all the permanent teeth.

EVALUATION OF ROENTGENOGRAM

It is well known that there is a magnification factor in the shadow of the tooth which is cast upon the x-ray film. For this reason direct measurement of images taken from the film will be somewhat greater than the measurement of the tooth itself. The degree of magnification depends upon the target-object distance and the object film distance. It is necessary to compensate for these factors if an accurate reading is to be made. If one can assume that the degree of magnification is approximately the same for the primary tooth as for its underlying permanent successor tooth can be calculated with close practical limits. Of course it is necessary to have sharp images on the film and freedom from overlapped contacts and rotations. The procedure for making this calculation is as follows:

Measure the width of the primary tooth on the x- ray film (Y') and the width of its underlying permanent successor (X') on the x- ray film. **(Figure 20)**

1. Measure the primary tooth (Y) directly in the mouth or on the orthodontic cast. **(Figure 21)**

2. The width of the unerupted permanent tooth(X) can then be calculated by a simple mathematical proportion

$$\frac{X}{X'} = \frac{Y}{Y'} \qquad \text{OR} \qquad X = \frac{X'Y}{Y'}$$

This procedure is followed for the three permanent successors on the right side, and the same for the left side. The two sides are compared and the results for each side should agree closely unless an anomaly is present. This information will then enable the dentist to evaluate the probability more closely.

- Huckaba developed a method for overcoming the effect of radiographic distortions while measuring the permanent canines and premolars MD width, using an equation relating the measures of erupted teeth to their radiographic images in order to obtain the proportional dimensions of unerupted teeth, as follows:[42]

$$\frac{x - Ray\ MD\ width\ of\ deciduous}{x - Ray\ MD\ width\ of\ the\ permanent} \times \frac{Real\ MD\ width\ of\ deciduous}{Real\ MD\ width\ of\ the\ permanent}$$

ADVANTAGE

- Can be used in maxillary and mandibular arches.

- Not require any prediction table.
- Very easy, practical and relatively accurate method.

LIMITATION

- Inherent distortion of radiographic image causes error.
- With respect to the random error, the method proposed by Huckaba was proven to be inadequate in terms of reproducibility, and should be used with caution to measure the required space in the mandibular arch. This suggests that care must be taken in borderline cases where the decision to extract or not teeth depends on meticulous analysis of the diagnostic elements.[42]
- More expensive.
- More time consuming.
- Require specific equipment.

CONCLUSION

Space analysis during mixed dentition is an important aspect to supervise the development of esthetics, functionally stable occlusion, and treatment planning. It implies preventive measures that are necessary to prevent a potential irregularity from progressing into severe malocclusion. The discrepancy between the space required and space available are common condition requiring early attention. While planning a treatment for such cases, it is of utmost importance to predict the deficiency in the arch space so that the indicated procedures could be performed as early as possible.

In the digital caliper method, systematic and random errors were considered acceptable. The brass wire measurement method did not present errors under the condition of repeatability; for reproducibility, however, the systematic error was significant and the random error indicates that this method should be considered inappropriate to measure space in the dental arch.[56]

Many methods of predicting the MD width of unerupted canines and premolars in the mixed dentition have been reported. These methods use three distinct ways to achieve their purposes. The first employs direct measurements of the teeth from radiographs with or without the use of a prediction formula as reported by Nance, Jensen et al. and Staley et al. The second uses prediction tables based on the measurements of other erupted permanent teeth, as reported by Ballard and Wylie, Carey, Moyers, Huckaba, Tanaka and Johnston, and Ferguson et al.[57]

There have been instances in which space maintaining appliances were placed in areas where space was already grossly inadequate, with the result that tooth extraction was necessary along with orthodontic space closure of the very space which was held open. The consequence, of course, was a needless appliance, an unnecessary expense, and a protraction of orthodontic treatment.[2]

The most accurate predictions of the mesio-distal widths of unerupted canines and premolars can be obtained by measurements of mesio-distal widths of these teeth on radiographs combined with measurement of mesio-distal widths of the erupted mandibular permanent teeth.[1] However; it requires the use of dental casts and radiographs to complete the analysis.[58]

TABLE1. PROBABILITY CHART FOR PREDICTING THE SUM OF WIDTHS OF $\underline{345}$ FROM $\overline{21/12}$

$\Sigma\ \overline{21/12}$	19.5	20.0	20.5	21.0	21.5	22.0	22.5	23.0	23.5	24.0	24.5	25.0	25.5	26.0	26.5	27.0
95%	21.1	21.4	21.7	22.0	22.3	22.6	22.9	25.2	25.3	24.1	24.4	24.7	25.0	25.3	25.6	25.8
85%	20.5	20.8	21.1	21.4	21.7	22.0	22.3	22.6	22.9	25.2	23.5	25.8	24.0	24.3	24.6	24.9
75%	20.1	20.4	20.7	23.0	21.3	21.6	21.3	22.2	22.3	22.8	25.1	23.4	23.7	24.0	24.3	24.5
65%	19.8	20.1	20.4	20.7	21.0	21.3	21.5	21.9	22.2	22.5	22.8	23.1	23.4	25.7	24.0	24.3
50%	19.4	19.7	2.0	20.3	20.6	20.9	21.2	21.5	21.8	22.1	22.4	22.7	25.0	25.5	25.6	25.9
35%	19.0	19.5	19.6	19.9	20.0	20.5	20.6	21.1	21.4	21.7	22.0	22.5	22.6	22.9	23.2	23.5
25%	18.7	19.0	19.3	19.6	19.9	20.2	20.5	20.5	21.1	21.4	21.7	22.0	22.3	22.6	22.9	25.2
15%	18.4	15.7	19.0	19.3	19.5	19.6	20.1	20.4	20.7	21.0	21.3	21.6	21.9	22.2	22.5	22.8
5%	17.7	18.0	18.3	18.6	18.0	19.0	19.5	19.8	20.1	20.4	20.7	21.0	21.3	21.6	21.9	22.2

TABLE 2: PROBABILITY CHART FOR PREDICTING THE SUM OF WIDTHS OF 345 FROM $\overline{21/12}$

Σ $\overline{21/12}$	19.5	20.0	20.5	21.0	21.5	22.0	22.5	23.0	23.5	24.0	24.5	25.0	25.5	26.0	26.5	27.0
95%	21.6	21.8	22.1	22.4	22.7	22.9	23.2	23.5	23.8	24.0	24.3	24.6	24.9	25.1	25.4	25.7
85%	21.0	21.3	21.5	21.8	22.1	22.4	22.6	22.9	23.2	23.5	23.7	24.0	24.3	24.6	24.8	25.1
75%	20.6	20.9	21.2	21.5	21.8	22.0	22.3	22.6	22.9	23.1	23.4	23.7	24.0	24.2	24.5	24.8
65%	20.4	20.6	20.9	21.2	21.5	21.8	22.0	22.3	22.6	22.8	23.1	23.4	23.7	24.0	24.2	24.5
50%	20.0	20.3	20.6	20.8	21.1	21.4	21.7	21.9	22.2	22.5	22.8	23.0	23.3	23.6	23.9	24.1
35%	19.6	19.9	20.2	20.5	20.8	21.0	21.3	21.6	21.9	22.1	22.4	22.7	23.0	23.2	23.5	23.8
25%	19.4	19.7	19.9	20.2	20.5	20.8	21.0	21.3	21.6	21.9	22.1	22.4	22.7	23.0	23.2	23.5
15%	19.0	19.3	19.6	19.9	20.2	20.4	20.7	21.0	21.3	21.5	21.8	22.1	22.4	22.6	22.9	23.2
5%	18.5	18.8	19.0	19.3	19.6	19.9	20.1	20.4	20.7	21.0	20.7	21.5	21.8	22.1	22.3	22.6

INGERVALL & LENNARTSON ANALYSIS

The possibility of predicting the breadths of unerupted canines and premolars is important in the supervision of the development of the dentition. Lack of space implies crowding and indicates that treatment will be necessary. Early prediction of lack of space facilitates treatment so that serial extraction can be started.

Various methods have been used for estimating the breadths of unerupted permanent canines and premolars:

1. Roentgenographic breadths of the unerupted teeth
2. Mean breadth of teeth
3. The breadth of the canine and premolars as judged from the total breadth of the lower incisors.

The first method has disadvantage that the image is somewhat enlarged and also that the tooth germ may be rotated with the result that the roentgenogram will give a false impression of its breadth.

The second method implies a serious risk of misjudging the space available after eruption of the teeth since the sum of the breadths of the canine and the premolar varies between 19 and 25mm. It is true that the mean value can be modified if the permanent teeth (incisors and first molars) already erupted are large, but the method is inexact.

Therefore several textbooks recommend the third method which is based on the intraindividual correlation in tooth size.

A combination of the breadths of the roentogenographic images of lower premolars and the breadths of erupted lower incisors as a basis for estimation of the breadth of the lower canine and premolars has been recommended by Hixon and Oldfather. They found such a combination to permit better prediction than methods previously available, but their method has apparently not found wide use.

Since the possibility of predicting the breadths of unerupted canines and premolars is clinically important and since such prediction can probably be improved by the combination of different predictors, it was considered of interest to try modifications of the method used by Hixon and Oldfather.

The best predictors can be readily selected with the use of stepwise multiple regression.

AIM

The purpose of this analysis was to investigate, with the aid of multiple regression, that which parameters of the mixed dentition were most useful for predicting the breadths of unerupted canines and premolars.

ARMAMENTARIUM

Stone casts

Intra-oral radiographs

Sliding calipers

Caliper compass

Transverse scale

PROCEDURE

A sample consisted of 77 children (38 boys and 39 girls) aged 9 years 1 month to 10 years 10 months. When the children were first seen the first permanent molars and permanent incisors had erupted to occlusion, while the permanent canines and premolars were unerupted.

On first examination alginate impression of both jaws were taken

↓

Stone casts were made

↓

Intra oral radiographs were obtained of permanent canines and premolars, from right side in 38 children and left side in the 39 children by using a modified bisecting angle technique.

↓

To obtain an orthoradial projection three intraoral roentgenograms were taken of the canine, first premolar and second premolar.

↓

Measurements were made with a caliper compass and a transverse scale

↓

Then Mesio-distal breadth of each first permanent molar and incisors were measured on the casts and bucco-lingual width of first permanent molar.

↓

The mesiodistal breadth was measured between the anatomic contact points, parallel to the occlusal plane. The buccolingual breadth was measured as the maximal distance between the buccal and the lingual surfaces perpendicular to the mesiodistal diameter of the tooth and parallel to the occlusal plane, if necessary down to the border of gingival on the cast.

↓

Mesiodistal breadths of crowns of the permanent canines and premolars were measured in the roentgenograms

↓

All measurements were made to the nearest tenth of a millimeter with well ground sliding calipers

↓

When all permanent canines and premolars had erupted to occlusion, new casts were made and mesio-distal width of canine and premolar was measured.

Roentgenograms were also used for estimating the degree of rotation of the unerupted premolars. The rotation of the premolars was estimated from the distance between the buccal and lingual cusps. The distance between the tips of the cusps perpendicular to the longitudinal axis of the tooth was measured. If the distance was 0-1mm, the degree of rotation was said to be 1; if 1.1-2.0mm, 2; and if it was more than 2.0mm, the degree of rotation was said to be 3. Rotation of degree 1 was most common (150 teeth) followed by degree 2 and degree 3 rotation among the various sorts of teeth given in table 1.

TABLE I

Distribution of teeth with rotation degrees 2 and 3.

	Degree of rotation	
Tooth	*2*	*3*
5+5	19	18
4+4	26	19
5—5	21	19
4—4	25	11

- The breadths of the individual teeth in the original casts and of the canine and premolars

in the radiograph were used as predictors for the mesio-distal of the permanent canine and premolars.

- The total breadth of the upper and lower incisors respectively also used as predictors. • In step 1 the program used selects the predictor variable with the greatest value for prediction of the dependent variable and step 2 and subsequent steps the next most useful variable. Since the regression is linear, a multiple normal distribution is presumed for statistical test.

RESULTS:

The sizes of teeth in the casts are given in table

Upper permanent teeth	M	S.D.	Range	Lower permanent teeth	M	S.D.	Range
Mesio-distal							
First molar	10.6	0.5	9.3-11.9	First molar	11.3	0.7	9.7-13.0
Second premolar	6.9	0.4	5.3-7.7	Second premolar	7.4	0.4	6.5-8.5
First premolar	7.2	0.4	6.2-8.3	First premolar	7.3	0.4	6.3-8.4
Canine	8.0	0.5	7.1-9.0	Canine	7.0	0.4	6.1-8.1
Lateral incisor	7.0	0.6	5.0-8.4	Lateral incisor	6.2	0.3	5.6-7.3
Central incisor	9.0	0.6	7.5-10.4	Central incisor	5.6	0.3	4.9-6.3
Bucco-lingual							
First molar	11.6	0.6	10.2-13.1	First molar	10.8	0.5	9.6-11.7
Total mesio-distal breadth							
Upper incisors	32.0	2.1	27.2-37.0	Lower incisors	23.6	1.1	21.4-26.8
Upper canine and premolars	22.0	1.0	19.7-24.7	Lower canine and premolars	21.6	0.9	19.4-23.5

Mean (M), standard deviation (S.D.), and range of variation in mm of breadths of teeth measured on casts of 77 children. Right and left sides pooled and sexes combined.

1. In the prediction of the breadth of an individual, unerupted permanent canine or premolar, the breadth of the homologous tooth invariably proved best.
2. The determination coefficient,(R^2) shows that about half of the variance in breadth of the upper second premolar can be explained by the breadth of the homologus tooth.
3. While three forths of the variance in breadth of the lower second premolar can be explained by the breadth of the homologus tooth.

Determination coefficients (R^2) in prediction of mesiodistal breadth of permanent canines and premolars with the breadth of the homologous tooth.

Upper tooth	R^2	*Lower tooth*	R^2
Second premolar	0.52	Second premolar	0.76
First premolar	0.72	First premolar	0.70
Canine	0.86	Canine	0.81

4. With three predictors it is possible to explain 62% of the variance of the total breadth of the upper canine and premolars. The regression equation is as follows: **(equation 1)**

- Total breadth of upper canine and premolars=4.77+0.55× buccolingual breadth of upper first molar+0.73×roentgenographic breadth of upper first premolar +0.58× roentgenographic breadth of upper canine.
- For the euqation the standard error of estimate about the regression line is 0.65mm.

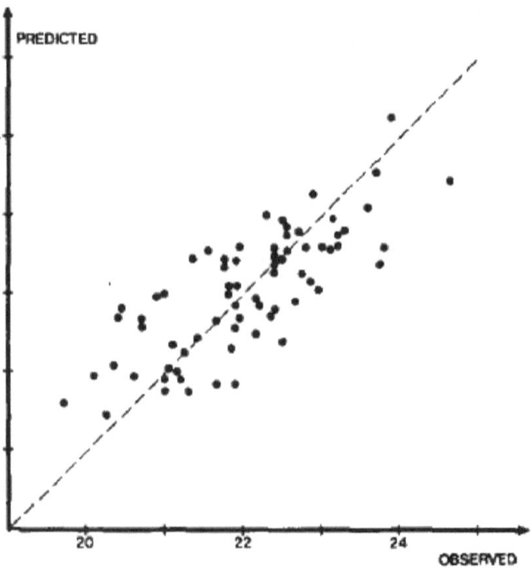

Fig. 1 Agreement between observed values of the total breadth of the upper canine and premolars and values predicted with equation 1. For an observed value (x-axis) the corresponding predicted value can be read on the y-axis.

Figure 1 compares the the oberved values of the total breadth of the upper canine and premolars and the values calculated from the equation. It is clear that the agreement between the observed and the calculated values was relatively good over the entire range of variation. The calculated values, however, tended to be too small in the upper part of the range of variation of the dependent variable and somewhat too large in the lower.

- When equation 1 was used the residuals in a probability plot showed a good normal distribution

5. If cases with rotation degree 3 of unerupted upper premolars are excluded, the regression equation is: **(equation 2)**

- Total breath of upper canine and premolars=2.5+1.23× roentgenographic breadth of upper first premolar+0.5×buccolingual breadth of upper first molar+0.55× roentgenographic breadth of upper second premolar.
- For the equation the standard error of estimate about the regresssion line is 0.59mm.
- The equation explains 72 percent of the variance of the total breadth of the upper canine and premolars.
- The residuals showed a fair normal distribution.

6. The measurements of the roentogram breadths of the unerupted teeth can explain 78 percent of the variance of the total breadth of the lower canine and premolars. The regression equation is: **(equation 3)**

- Total breath of upper canine and premolars=4.49+1.14× roentgenographic breadth of lower first premolar+0.62×buccolingual breadth of lower canine+0.47× roentgenographic breadth of lower second premolar.
- The standard of error of estimate about the regression line is 0.45mm.
- The probablity plot of residuals showed a good normal distribution.

7. If the upper and lower first premolars have erupted so their mesiodistal bredths can be measured, it is possible to predict three forths of the total breadth of the canines and the premolars solely with the first premolar as predictor. The determinant coefficient was 0.76 for the upper jaw and 0.73 for the lower and the regression quations: **(equation 4)**

- Total breath of upper canine and premolars=6.25+2.19× measiodistal breadth of upper first premolar.
- The standard errror of estimate about the regresssion line was 0.49mm.
- Probability plot of residuals showed a good normal distribution.

8. Total breadth of lower canine and premolars=7.15+1.99×measiodistal breadth of lower first premolar. **(equation 5)**

- The standard errror of estimate about the regresssion line was 0.49mm.
- Probability plot of residuals showed a good normal distribution.

Comparison between the observed values and those calculated from equations 4 and 5 revealed no systematic devaition for any part of the range of variation. A probability plot of the residuals showed a good normal distribution whether equation 4 or 5 was used.[15]

CONCLUSION:

- The sizes of the teeth were identical to those in other swedish series. The material may therefore regarded as representative of the swedish population.
- No endeavour was made to test decidous teeth as predictors since it has been weaker correlation than between the breaths of permanent teeth.[6]
- Since the material consisted of as many boys as girls, the regression equation holds for both sexes. Earlier investigations have also shown that the use of both sexes together is possible without impairment of the results in the calculation of correlations between the sizes of teeth.[11]
- If great accuracy is required in the prediction of the space available in the upper jaw, equation 1 can be used in patients with rotated unerupted teeth.

- At least three forth of variance of total breadth of canine and premolars can be explained by their measurement in radiographs. Hence equation 3 is prefered to use of mean value for the breadth of unerupted teeth.
- In the upper jaw first premolar usually erupts before canine and second premolar, if first premolar has been erupted, three forth of variance of total breadth of canine and premolar can be explained by the use of breadth of the first premolar as a predictor.
- In the lower jaw the canine often erupts earlier than premolars. The total breadth can then be predicted with aid of equation 5.
- Neither in the prediction of the total breadth of the upper nor lower premolars and canine was the total breadth of incisors of any significance.
- Results are different from hixon and oldfather method because they recommend combination consisting of radiographic breadths of canine and premolars and measurements on cast of the breadths of lower central and lateral incisors.
- This investigation shows that the best variables available as predictors in the early mixed dentition are the roentgenographic breadths of the teeth in question. This is in agreement with the conclusion of Moorrees and Reed and Arya et al. ,who showed that the correlations between the breadths of teeth measured on casts are too weak to be of any practical value for prediction.[11]

LEVERN MERRIFIED ANALYSIS

This analysis was developed by L. Levern Merrifield, Herbert A. Klontz, and James L. Vaden in the year 1978. They link clinical research to fundamental orthodontic concepts to give the clinician a workable differential diagnosis system. The clinical research, conducted by the Charles Tweed Foundation, attempted to establish a "profile" for the Class II malocclusion correction, which, because of certain characteristics, was destined to failure. The Cranial Facial Dental Analysis integrates this clinical research with the total space analysis to give the clinical orthodontist a useful tool for differential diagnosis.[20]

AIM /OBJECTIVE

Objective in preparing this differential diagnosis and clinical analysis was to incorporate the results of clinical research conducted by the Charles H. Tweed International Foundation for Orthodontic Research with time-tested concepts and values that significantly influence orthodontic diagnosis and the subsequent delivery of a quality orthodontic service to the public.

ARMAMENTARIUM

Pretreatment and post-treatment cephalometric x-ray films with tracings of specified cephalometric landmarks.

PROCEDURE

- Dr. Gramling compiled a large sample of successfully and unsuccessfully treated Class II malocclusions, all of which were treated by members of the Charles H. Tweed Foundation.[59]
- The clinical material used reflected treatment with the Sequential Directional Force technology that was introduced in 1978. All the data therefore represented similar technology and treatment strategy.

- Each member who participated in Dr. Gramling's studies furnished pretreatment and post-treatment cephalometric x-ray films with tracings of specified cephalometric landmarks.
- The points were then checked by Dr. Gramling for consistency of technique.
- The pretreatment and post-treatment Frankfort horizontal planes were standardized by means of superimposition on the sella nasion plane. Contributors were not handpicked; anyone who used the Sequential Directional Force technology was encouraged to participate.
- Dr. Gramling collected the "successful" sample and also collected a sample of 55 patients whose Class II malocclusions were deemed unsuccessfully corrected by the contributors. **(Figure 22)**
- The same statistical analyses were performed on the successful and unsuccessful samples.
- Many values were considered, but the values scrutinized most closely are illustrated in Fig. I.

RESULTS

The results of the studies of unsuccessful and successful treatment were compared and can be seen in Table 1

Table I. Comparison of successful and unsuccessful samples

	Successful		*Unsuccessful*	
	Pretreatment	*Posttreatment*	*Pretreatment*	*Posttreatment*
FMA	28	27	29	30
FMIA	58	63	56	61
IMPA	95	90	95	95
Z-angle	66	75	62	69
Y-Axis	62	62	65	65
SNA	82	79	82	79
SNB	76	76	75	75
ANB	6	3	6	4
AOBO	4	−1	7	5

In the successful sample,

- The Frankfort mandibular plane angle (FMA) was reduced,

- The Frankfort mandibular incisor angle (FMIA) was increased,
- The incisor mandibular plane angle (IMPA) was reduced

In the unsuccessful sample,

- FMA increased,
- FMIA increased but not as much as it did in the successful sample,
- IMPA remained the same.

There was not as much Z-angle increase in the unsuccessful sample as there was in the successful sample. The SNA angle reduction was similar, but AOBO reduction for the unsuccessful sample was not as good as for the successful sample. The Y-axis values and the SNB angle values remained the same for both samples.

Conclusion

By studying the collected data from these two samples, it can be concluded that in unsuccessful Class II treatment, the mandibular incisor position is not corrected, or if it is corrected, the correction is subsequently compromised by excessive, unreciprocated use of Class II elastics in an attempt to establish the proper anterior-posterior maxillomandibular relationships.

In the next comparison, the successful and unsuccessful treatment results were divided into high, medium, and low Frankfort mandibular plane angle categories (Table II).

Table II. Comparison of successful and unsuccessful samples by dividing the samples according to FMA

	Comparisons	
	Successful	*Unsuccessful*
Low Frankfort mandibular plane angle		
FMA	+1	+1
FMIA	+7	−1
IMPA	−6	0
ANB	−3	−2
Z-angle	+10	+8
Medium Frankfort mandibular plane angle		
FMA	+1	0
FMIA	+6	0
IMPA	−6	0
ANB	−3	−3
Z-angle	+10	+11
High Frankfort mandibular plane angle		
FMA	+1	0
FMIA	+4	−1
IMPA	−3	−1
ANB	−2	−1
Z-angle	+8	+6

According to the data from the low FMA category, the ANB angle changes were not much different between the groups. The big difference was in mandibular incisor position. In the successful orthodontic treatment sample, the mandibular incisors were uprighted more than in the unsuccessful sample

The FMIA was increased 8° more in the successful sample than in the unsuccessful sample. Thus, facial change was more positive in the successful sample.

In the medium Frankfort mandibular plane angle category, unsuccessful treatment was about equal to successful treatment, except the mandibular incisors were uprighted more in the successful sample of patients. An analysis of the high angle category showed similar results.

- The Class II malocclusion was successfully corrected when:
    1) The FMA was maintained,
    2) The FMIA increased,
    3) The IMPA decreased,
    4) The ANB angle reduced.

- Class II malocclusion whose treatment can lead to failure, in which following parameters are present:
    1) A very high or very low FMA,
    2) A high ANB angle,
    3) A high AO/BO,
    4) A low FMIA or a high IMPA,
    5) A steep occlusal plane angle,
    6) A very low SNB angle.

PROBABILITY INDEX

From the background of evidence established by these studies, Gramling formulated a "Probability Index' for three specific purposes [60]

(1) To augment diagnostic procedures,

(2) To guide treatment procedures, and

(3) To predict possible treatment success or failure.

- The purpose of the index was to be of value in isolating those Class II malocclusions that might need alternate treatment procedures or those that might require surgical procedures to affect a complete correction.
- Gramling's probability index was based on the premise that control of the FMA, the ANB angle, the FMIA, the occlusal plane, and the SNB angle were keys to the success or failure of the orthodontic treatment of a Class II malocclusion.
- The Probability Index suggested that the following conditions might be necessary for treatment success of a Class II malocclusion:

    1. The FMA should be 18° to 35°.
    2. The ANB angle should be 6° or less.
    3. The FMIA should be greater than 60°.
    4. The occlusal plane should be 7° or less.
    5. The SNB angle should be 80° or more.

- Gramling established a difficulty factor and assigned a specific number of points to each variable (Table III A).

Table IIIA. Difficulty factors—weighted variables of the probability index

Probability index variables	
FMA:	Variation - 5 points
ANB:	Variation - 15 points
FMIA:	Variation - 2 points
OcPl:	Variation - 3 points
SNB:	Variation - 5 points

In 1989 Gramling studied 40 successful and 40 unsuccessful Class II malocclusion corrections. After studying these 80 patient records, he revised only one of the five premises of the Probability Index. He changed the successful the FMA range from 18°-35° to 22°-28° (Table IIIB).

Table IIIB. The probability index

	Point value	*Cephalometric value*	*Probability index*
FMA 22°-28°	5		
ANB 6 or less	15		
FMIA 60 or more	2		
OCC PL 7 or less	3		
SNB 80 or more	5		
		Total	______

In a later study of successful and unsuccessful Class II treatment, Merrifield and Gebeck' studied a successfully treated Class II sample, an unsuccessfully treated Class II sample, and a control Class II sample. As a result of their studies, Merrifield and Gebeck concluded that equally important to successful Class II correction was control of anterior facial height and posterior facial height, or as Gramling concluded by using FMA and occlusal plane, control of the vertical dimension.

Posterior facial height is a millimetric measurement of ramus height from articulare to the mandibular plane which is measured tangent to the posterior border of the ramus. Anterior facial height used by Merrifield and Gebeck is a perpendicular millimetric measurement from palatal plane to menton.

The relationship of posterior facial height to anterior facial height determines both the FMA and the lower face proportion. In Class II treatment, it is essential to limit the increase in anterior facial height by controlling maxillary and mandibular molar extrusion and by using an anterior high-pull force on the maxilla.

Merrifield and Gebeck stated that the ratio of change of posterior facial height to anterior facial height was a very valuable evaluation tool both during and after orthodontic treatment. They found that a ratio of two times as much posterior facial height increase as anterior facial height increase was ideal for Class II, Division 1 malocclusion correction and for dento-alveolar protrusion reduction.[20]

In 1989, Andre Horn studied and researched the relationship of anterior and posterior facial height. Horn suggested a Facial Height Index or FHI. The normal posterior facial height to anterior facial height ratio was found by Horn to be 0.65 to 0.75. If the FHI value was below or above this range, the malocclusion was a great deal more complex and the difficulty encountered in correction was increased.[62]

CRANIAL FACIAL ANALYSIS

The Cranial Facial Analysis has been developed from Gramling's work, from Merrifield and Gebeck's work, and from Andre Horn's ratio studies.

When the cranial facial analysis is used in conjunction with the total dentition space analysis, the clinician can determine the complexity of the major clinical aspects of a malocclusion. Use of both analyses will significantly improve the clinician's ability to diagnose, plan, and execute treatment.

The total space analysis (TSA) was developed by **Levern Marrifield (1978).**

This method was divided into three areas. Anterior middle and posterior and the resulting values for each area were added together to yield the final deficit.

FMA - Frankfort mandibular plane angle

FMPA – Incisor mandibular plane angle

FMIA – Frankfort mandibular incisor angle

Anterior area: For this area the calculation of the difference between space required and space available was done as before. [Using tooth dimension and brass ligature wire].

Tooth measurement: Measurements of mandibular incisor widths on the casts were added to the values obtained from the radiographic measurements of the canine.

Cephalometric Correction: The actual FMIA (in degrees) is subtracted from proposed angle and the difference (in degrees) is multiplied by a constant (O.S) to give the difference in millimeters.

Soft tissue modification: The soft tissue modification was derived by measuring the 'Z' angle of Merrifield and adding Cephalometric correction (in degrees) to it. If the corrected Z angle is greater than 80^0 the mandibular incisor inclination was modified as necessary (upto an IMPA of approximately 92^0). If the corrected angle was less than 75^0, additional up righting of incisor is necessary.

Upper lip thickness was measured from the vermilion border of the lip to the greatest curvature of the labial surface of central incisor.

Total chin thickness was measured from the soft tissue chin to the N-B line. If the lip thickness is greater than chin thickness, the difference in mm is determined by multiplying by 2 and adding it to the space required. If it is less than or equal to chin thickness, no soft tissue modification was necessary.

Middle area: In this area calculations are made of the difference between space required and space available.

Tooth measurement: The crown widths of the permanent mandibular first molar are measured at their greatest mesiodistal diameter on the cast. These values are added to the measurements of the premolars obtained from the radiographs.

Curve of occlusion: The space required to level the mandibular curve of occlusion was determined. A flat object was placed on the occlusal surface of the mandibular teeth contacting the permanent first molars and the incisors. The deepest point between the flat surface and the occlusal surfaces of the primary molar is measured on both sides.

$$\text{Curve of occlusion formula} = \frac{\text{RT side depth} + \text{LT side depth}}{2} + 0.5\text{mm}$$

This value is added to tooth measurements. Space available was determined by placing two brass wires (0.033 inch) from the mesiobuccal line angle of permanent first molar on one side to the other side.

Posterior area: For this area determinations were made of the space required and space available. [49]

The space required consisted of sum of the mesiodistal widths of the two second and third molars. [Radiographic enlargement was calculated]. In cases where third molar is not visible wheeler's dimensions were used and calculation is as follows. [49]

$$x = \frac{y \cdot x^1}{y^1}$$

x = Estimated value of $\overline{8|}$

x^1 = Wheelers value of $\overline{8|}$

y = Actual size of $\overline{6|}$

y^1 = Wheelers value of $\overline{6|}$

Space available consisted of the space presently available plus the estimated increase or prediction. (The estimated increase was 3mm/yrs (1.5mm each side) until 14years age in girls and 16 yrs in boys).

Average linear change in position of lower third molar over the period of 5 years is 5.4mm.[63]

The amount of growth from the lower first molar to the anterior border of the ramus from 8 years to 14 years was 7.7 mm. The growth from 14 years to an average of the ages from 16 to 20 years was 2.3 mm. The growth from the lower first molar to the posterior border of the ramus was 6.6 mm from 8 to 14 years, while 2.5 mm growth occurred after that.[64]

The space needed was obtained by measuring the distance on the occlusal plane between perpendiculars drawn from the occlusal plane tangent to the distal surface of permanent first molar to the anterior border of the ramus on the lateral Cephalometric tracing.[49]

CRANIAL FACIAL ANALYSIS	Ceph	Difficulty	
Normal Range	Value	Factor	Difficulty
FMA 22° - 28°	____	5	____
ANB 1° - 5°	____	15	____
Z Angle 70° - 80°	____	2	____
Occ Plane 8° - 12°	____	3	____
SNB 78° - 82°	____	5	____
FHI (PFH:AFH) .65 - .75	____	3	____
C.F. Difficulty Total			____

TOTAL SPACE ANALYSIS			
		Difficulty	
Anterior	Value	Factor	Difficulty
Tooth Arch Disc.	____	1.5	____
Headfilm Disc.	____	1	____
Soft Tissue Mod.	____	.5	____
TOTAL	____		____
Midarch			
Tooth Arch Disc.	____		
Curve of Spee	____		
TOTAL	____	1	____
Occlusal Disharmony			
(Class II or Class III) ____		2	____
Posterior			
Tooth Arch Disc.	____		
Expected Increase (-)	____		
TOTAL	____	.5	____
Space Analysis Total	____	Space Analysis Difficulty Total	____

The total space analysis developed by Merrifield took into account the tooth measurement, cephalometric correction and soft tissue modification. This method also indicated the exact area (anterior, middle or posterior) where the crowding occurred.[25]

[2] PREDICTION BASED ON MEASUREMENTS OF ALREADY ERUPTED PERMANENT TEETH-ON DENTAL CASTS

SEIPEL ANALYSIS

This method was recommended by Carl Michael Seipel in 1946. This method was based upon the estimation of size of permanent canine and premolar by prediction based on measurements of already erupted permanent teeth on dental casts.

AIM

Seipel attempted to predict the mesio-distal width of mandibular permanent canine and premolar teeth based on the mesio-distal width of the corresponding mandibular central incisor. The correlation coefficient was found to be low in all three cases.[8]

ARMAMENTARIUM

- Dental cast
- Boley gauge
- Millimeter ruler

PROCEDURE

- Seipel measured the:
  1. Sizes of separate teeth,
  2. The position of the teeth,
  3. The orientation of the dentition to adjacent parts of the skull.
- Included were such measurements as transverse dimensions of the dental arch, length of the dental arch, and inter maxillary relations.
- These measurements were taken on the following three age groups:
  1. Aged 4 years;
  2. Aged 13 years;
  3. Aged 21 years.
- Both males and females were examined.
- Sex differences were found with regard to tooth form, jaw size, and to some extent also in tooth position with variations being more pronounced in the age groups from 13 to 21 years.

TABLE I. TOOTH SIZE, MESIODISTAL WIDTH IN MM.

Mean Values of Right and Left Side. No. = Number of Individuals Examined. $M \pm \epsilon(M)$ = Arithmetical Mean ± Standard Error of the Mean. σ = Standard Deviation.

TEETH	TEMPORARY DENTITION						PERMANENT DENTITION					
	MALES			FEMALES			MALES			FEMALES		
	NO.	$M \pm \epsilon(M)$	σ	NO.	$M \pm \epsilon(M)$	σ	NO.	$M \pm \epsilon(M)$	σ	NO.	$M \pm \epsilon(M)$	σ
Upper Jaw												
I_1	205	6.60 ± 0.028	0.41	203	6.56 ± 0.027	0.38	483	8.84 ± 0.025	0.55	490	8.62 ± 0.024	0.53
I_2	224	5.46 ± 0.023	0.35	236	5.36 ± 0.024	0.37	469	6.81 ± 0.028	0.60	476	6.64 ± 0.026	0.57
C	249	7.04 ± 0.025	0.40	250	6.93 ± 0.019	0.30	463	8.10 ± 0.020	0.46	473	7.73 ± 0.019	0.41
P_1	88	7.31 ± 0.041	0.39	85	7.18 ± 0.042	0.38	135	7.18 ± 0.033	0.38	124	7.04 ± 0.035	0.39
P_2	124	8.94 ± 0.044	0.49	120	8.79 ± 0.037	0.40	125	6.97 ± 0.035	0.39	115	6.85 ± 0.040	0.43
M_1							164	10.69 ± 0.038	0.48	135	10.47 ± 0.045	0.52
M_2							151	10.47 ± 0.053	0.65	176	10.05 ± 0.044	0.58
M_3							33	9.48 ± 0.170	0.98	7	8.33	
Σ Inc.		24.05 ± 0.051			23.82 ± 0.051			31.25 ± 0.075			30.45 ± 0.072	
$I_1 + I_2 + C$		19.10 ± 0.044			18.85 ± 0.041			23.75 ± 0.043			22.99 ± 0.040	
$I_1 - P_2$		35.35 ± 0.075			34.82 ± 0.069			37.90 ± 0.064			36.88 ± 0.067	
$I_1 - M_2$								59.06 ± 0.092			57.40 ± 0.092	
Height I_1	237	5.52 ± 0.037	0.57	240	5.43 ± 0.035	0.55	255	9.68 ± 0.054	0.87	243	9.32 ± 0.057	0.88
Lower Jaw												
I_1	242	4.25 ± 0.020	0.32	241	4.16 ± 0.016	0.25	507	5.51 ± 0.016	0.36	491	5.42 ± 0.017	0.37
I_2	247	4.86 ± 0.022	0.35	248	4.81 ± 0.020	0.32	507	6.13 ± 0.018	0.40	493	5.94 ± 0.017	0.37
C	250	6.04 ± 0.029	0.32	250	5.92 ± 0.021	0.33	503	7.12 ± 0.017	0.39	493	6.69 ± 0.017	0.38
P_1	124	8.00 ± 0.041	0.46	123	7.85 ± 0.037	0.41	160	7.27 ± 0.029	0.37	146	7.16 ± 0.033	0.40
P_2	136	9.94 ± 0.041	0.48	151	9.80 ± 0.041	0.51	103	7.41 ± 0.040	0.41	117	7.21 ± 0.036	0.39
M_1							145	11.24 ± 0.047	0.57	123	10.98 ± 0.055	0.61
M_2							241	11.15 ± 0.041	0.69	275	10.70 ± 0.039	0.64
M_3							52	11.32 ± 0.120	0.84	11	10.30	
Σ Inc.		18.22 ± 0.041			17.96 ± 0.037			23.24 ± 0.046			22.59 ± 0.047	
$I_1 + I_2 + C$		15.15 ± 0.036			14.89 ± 0.033			18.47 ± 0.029			18.05 ± 0.029	
$I_1 - P_2$		33.09 ± 0.068			32.54 ± 0.064			33.44 ± 0.058			32.42 ± 0.057	
$I_1 - M_2$								55.83 ± 0.086			54.10 ± 0.088	
Height I_1	243	4.98 ± 0.033	0.52	242	4.88 ± 0.031	0.48	255	8.33 ± 0.051	0.82	243	8.21 ± 0.046	0.71

TABLE II. VARIATIONS OF TOOTH-SIZE (MES.-DIST. CROWN-WIDTH) IN THE PERMANENT DENTITION
Variations Expressed in Arithmetic Mean (= M) and Standard Deviation (= σ).

TEETH		MEAN	M - σ						M + σ					
			-3σ	-2.5σ	-2σ	-1.5σ	$-\sigma$	-0.5σ	$+0.5\sigma$	$+\sigma$	$+1.5\sigma$	$+2\sigma$	$+2.5\sigma$	$+3\sigma$
Males Upper jaw	I_1	8.84	7.19	7.46	7.74	8.01	8.29	8.56	9.12	9.39	9.67	9.94	10.22	10.49
	I_2	6.81	5.01	5.31	5.61	5.91	6.21	6.51	7.11	7.41	7.71	8.01	8.31	8.61
	C	8.10	6.72	6.95	7.18	7.41	7.64	7.87	8.33	8.56	8.79	9.02	9.25	9.48
	P_1	7.18	6.04	6.23	6.42	6.61	6.80	6.99	7.37	7.56	7.75	7.94	8.13	8.32
	P_2	6.97	5.80	5.99	6.19	6.38	6.58	6.77	7.17	7.36	7.56	7.75	7.95	8.14
	M_1	10.69	9.25	9.49	9.73	9.97	10.21	10.45	10.93	11.17	11.41	11.65	11.89	12.13
	M_2	10.47	8.52	8.84	9.17	9.49	9.82	10.14	10.80	11.12	11.45	11.77	12.10	12.42
Lower jaw	I_1	5.51	3.92	4.18	4.45	4.71	4.98	5.24	5.78	6.04	6.31	6.57	6.84	7.10
	I_2	6.13	4.42	4.70	4.99	5.27	5.56	5.84	6.42	6.70	6.99	7.27	7.56	7.84
	C	7.12	5.89	6.09	6.30	6.50	6.71	6.91	7.33	7.53	7.74	7.94	8.15	8.35
	P_1	7.27	6.10	6.29	6.49	6.68	6.88	7.07	7.47	7.66	7.86	8.05	8.25	8.44
	P_2	7.41	6.12	6.33	6.55	6.76	6.98	7.19	7.63	7.84	8.06	8.27	8.49	8.70
	M_1	11.24	9.68	9.94	10.20	10.46	10.72	10.98	11.50	11.76	12.02	12.28	12.54	12.80
	M_2	11.15	9.41	9.70	9.99	10.28	10.57	10.86	11.44	11.73	12.02	12.31	12.60	12.89
Females Upper jaw	I_1	8.62	7.54	7.72	7.90	8.08	8.26	8.44	8.80	8.98	9.16	9.34	9.52	9.70
	I_2	6.64	5.44	5.64	5.84	6.04	6.24	6.44	6.84	7.04	7.24	7.44	7.64	7.84
	C	7.73	6.56	6.75	6.95	7.14	7.34	7.53	7.93	8.12	8.32	8.51	8.71	8.90
	P_1	7.01	5.93	6.11	6.30	6.48	6.67	6.85	7.23	7.41	7.60	7.78	7.97	8.15
	P_2	6.85	5.62	5.82	6.03	6.23	6.44	6.64	7.06	7.26	7.47	7.67	7.88	8.08
	M_1	10.47	8.76	9.04	9.33	9.61	9.90	10.18	10.76	11.04	11.33	11.61	11.90	12.18
	M_2	10.05	7.98	8.32	8.67	9.01	9.36	9.70	10.40	10.74	11.09	11.43	11.78	12.12
Lower jaw	I_1	5.42	4.31	4.49	4.68	4.86	5.05	5.23	5.61	5.79	5.98	6.16	6.35	6.53
	I_2	5.94	4.83	5.01	5.20	5.38	5.57	5.75	6.13	6.31	6.50	6.68	6.87	7.05
	C	6.69	5.55	5.74	5.93	6.12	6.31	6.50	6.88	7.07	7.27	7.45	7.64	7.83
	P_1	7.16	5.96	6.16	6.36	6.56	6.76	6.96	7.36	7.56	7.76	7.96	8.16	8.36
	P_2	7.21	6.04	6.23	6.43	6.62	6.82	7.01	7.41	7.60	7.80	7.99	8.19	8.38
	M_1	10.98	9.15	9.45	9.76	10.06	10.37	10.67	11.29	11.59	11.90	12.20	12.51	12.81
	M_2	10.70	8.78	9.17	9.42	9.73	10.06	10.38	11.02	11.34	11.62	11.98	12.23	12.62

RESULTS/ FINDINGS

- It was found that there is a pronounced positive correlation with regard to the size of teeth in the same jaw with the different component varying in the same direction in relation to the mean value. Individuals with large incisors also have other teeth of larger than average size.

- With regard to variations of tooth position in the dental arch, as can be observed clinically from the crowns of the teeth, it appears that such variations are mainly in the form of spacing, rotations, proximal contact alterations, and changes following the loss of teeth.
- In the deciduous dentition, spacing predominates while crowding is to be found more frequently in the permanent dentition. The frequency of spacing is higher in the upper jaw while crowding appears more frequently in the lower jaw.
- In the deciduous dentition spacing is comparatively evenly distributed. At the age of 4 years the maxilla shows minimum spacing especially about the canine region which has been called a primate type of spacing. In the permanent dentition, spacing is usually localized between the canines and first premolar and between the second central incisors in the upper jaw.
- Crowding in the adult permanent dentition is to be found in the third molar region. Anterior to the first molars crowding is found in the deciduous dentition about the incisor and canine regions.
- In the early permanent dentition, crowding is usually to be observed in the canine regions of the maxillary jaw and is more pronounced in males than in females.
- In the mandibular jaw, crowding is more often localized about the second premolar and incisors. Crowding about the lower second premolars is more common in males than in females. An observation is made about such mandibular crowding that it appears to be a transitional phenomenon which is considerably reduced in the 21-year group. Mandibular canines and incisors, on the other hand, show a tendency to increase in crowding as age increases.
- The most frequent sites for crowding are given as follows:
  At age 4 years minimum crowding and rotation of the mandibular incisor region;
  At age 13 years crowding of the later erupting permanent teeth;
  At age 21 years increasing crowding of the anterior region especially of the mandibular jaw.

- Rotation of teeth is usually concomitant of crowding but occurs also in cases where the space usually allotted for a tooth is so large as to interfere with proximal contact. While rotations occur in 4 per cent of deciduous dentitions, it is to be observed in almost 15 per cent of permanent dentitions.
- Changes in the position of the teeth following extraction confirm Salz-Mann's findings published in 1938. It was shown at that time that second molar teeth adjacent to extracted first molars migrate forward especially in the maxillary jaw, while the premolars show distal migration especially in the lower jaw. There is a distal migration of anterior teeth with an increase of spacing and a decrease of crowding. The dental migration is more pronounced in the lower jaw.
- Closure of space in the deciduous dentition is slow while in the permanent dentition it is faster and more definite. While only 10 per cent of the spaces in the deciduous dentitions are found to close fully, 50 per cent of the spaces in the permanent dentitions show closure. A pronounced correlation was found between molar and incisor relations. Jaw malocclusions are found to be less frequent than malocclusions due to arch relationship. The significant factor is that intermaxillary relationship is of a stable, individual character which tends to be maintained during tooth change and jaw growth.

CONCLUSION

In conclusion, Seipel shows that while frequent positional variations of spacing and crowding appear in size-space, disturbances there are also specific from variations which appear independent of available space in the jaws.

Seipel has presented an account of variations of tooth position and tooth size which will be found of value to workers in the field of orthodontic research as well as to practicing orthodontists. His findings are an extremely valuable contribution to the orthodontic literature.

- Seipel made all of his measurements of the deciduous and permanent teeth directly, without resorting to impressions and casts.

- Seipel 's findings on mesiodistal crown diameters of Swedes are the data that furnish sufficient statistics for comparative studies dealing with populations of white stock.
- The mean mesiodistal crown diameters of the deciduous teeth are smaller for the North American children studied by Moorreess than for the Swedish children measured by Seipel except in the case of the deciduous maxillary second molars.[11]
- The children studied by Seipel have a larger mesiodistal diameter of the tooth crowns than those studied by Lundstr6m, except in the case of the mandibular lateral incisor of the boys (which is markedly smaller in Seipel's series than in that of Lundstrdm).[65]

BALLARD AND WYLIE ANALYSIS

This quantitative analysis was recommended by Murray L. Ballard and Wendell L. Wylie in the year 1947. They conducted an investigation to evaluate the assumption that there is harmony in tooth size in any one individual; that is, if the incisors are larger than average, the canines, premolars and molars are also correspondingly larger than average. This is a simple method of estimating the width of the mandibular canines, first premolar, and second premolar of one side from the total mesiodistal width of the four mandibular incisors.[9]

Ballard has shown that the dental arches are not the refined set of "gears" which some have thought them to be. He compared the mesiodistal widths of teeth of one side with those of corresponding teeth on the other side, and showed that in 90 per cent of the 500 cases examined, a discrepancy of a quarter of a millimeter or more could be found in one or more pairs of teeth, and that in 80 per cent of the cases this discrepancy amounted to half a millimeter or more. Clinical evidence lately adduced indicates that quantitative measurements may be profitably used in practice and applied at an earlier age than was therefore thought possible.[9]

The ease and accuracy with which Nance mixed dentition analysis is accomplished is greatly affected by the quality of the x-rays available for the orthodontist's use. The accuracy with which the mesiodistal widths of unerupted teeth may be determined depends in large part upon the technique with which the films were taken, but even when these variables are reduced to a minimum, teeth may be rotated in their crypts so that a true measurement of mesiodistal width cannot be determined from intraoral or extraoral films even when they are beyond reproach.[4]

The information provided in this report may be used as an adjunct to Nance's method of case analysis, or in any other situation which it is desirable to know the total mesiodistal width of unerupted canines and premolars.

ARMAMENTARIUM

- Dividers
- Millimeter rule
- Record card
- Plaster models

INCLUSION CRITERIA

- All permanent incisors, canines, premolars and first molars that were fully erupted
- All models are from plaster impression.

PROCEDURE

- Dentists have always assumed that there is some harmony in tooth size in one mouth, that is, if the incisors of a given individual are somewhat larger than the average, the canine premolars and molars in that person will be correspondingly larger than the average for those teeth.[16]
- In order to determine the extent of this consistency and to put it to use, the mesiodistal width of every mandibular tooth back to and including first permanent molars was obtained from plaster models by means of dividers and a millimeter rule, and recorded on a card for each of 441 individuals.

- No cases were included in the series unless all permanent incisors, canines, premolars and first molars were fully erupted, permitting accurate measurement.
- All models were made from plaster impressions. Measurements were read to the nearest one-quarter millimeter.
- The sum of the four permanent mandibular incisors was determined for each individual, as was the sum of the canine, first premolar, and second premolar of one side.
- If there was found a discrepancy in mesiodistal width between right and left canines or premolars, a mean value was taken for the tooth in question.

RESULTS

- The mean sum of the four mandibular permanent incisors was 23.84 ± 0.08 millimeters.
- The mean sum of the canine, first premolar, and second premolar of one side was 21.97 ±0.06 millimeters.
- The mean width of mandibular first permanent molars was found to be 11.20 ± 0.03 millimeters.
- Still another value, the coefficient of correlation, must be calculated in order to determine, in a large group, the extent to which the sum of the canine, first premolar, and second premolar varies as the sum of the four incisors increases or decreases. The coefficient of correlation may vary from -1.0, which indicates a perfect inverse relationship between two variables, to +l.0, which indicates a perfect direct relationship between two variables. A coefficient of correlation of

0.0 indicates a completely chance relationship between the two variables in question.

- The coefficient of correlation between the sum of the four mandibular incisors and the sum of the canine, first premolar, and second premolar of one side was found to be +0.64.
- Once this coefficient of correlation has been determined, it is an easy matter to devise a formula whereby one may predict one of the variables when the other is known. This is the situation which we have in the mixed dentition, where the mandibular incisors and first permanent molars have erupted but where the mandibular canines and premolars are unerupted and therefore not susceptible to direct measurement of mesiodistal widths. The formula is as follows :

$$X = 9.41 + 0.527Y,$$

Where X equals the sum of the canine, first premolars, and second premolars of one side of the mandibular arch, and Y equals the sum of the four mandibular incisors.

In reality it is not necessary to make this calculation each time one seeks to determine the width of the three unerupted teeth in a mixed dentition case, since the device shown in Figure renders calculation unnecessary. **(Figure 24)**

One simply measures the four incisors (it is best to measure these teeth individually with dividers and prick the mesio-distal width of each tooth onto the same line of a lined card, so that the dividers may then be opened to make an accurate measurement of the sum of the four), determines the sum in millimeters by using an accurate rule, and finds this number on the left side of the scale in Figure. Directly opposite, on the right side of the scale, will be found the sum of the three unerupted teeth which may be expected for that case. Obviously, this value, derived as it is, is only an estimate of the sum of these teeth, the true sum of which can be determined only by direct measurement.

Since mandibular first permanent molars are fully erupted by the time the four incisors are available for measurement, the first permanent molars may be measured in a mixed dentition case as well. It is conceivable that when the measurement of the first permanent molars is combined with the sum of the mandibular incisors for predictive purposes, a more accurate value for the three unerupted teeth would be obtained. In order to test this, two other coefficients of correlation were determined.

The coefficient of correlation between the mesiodistal width of the first permanent molar and the sum of the canine and the premolars of one side was found to be +0.51. A coefficient of correlation between the mesiodistal width of the mandibular first permanent molar and the sum of the four mandibular incisors was found to be +0.47. These values were then worked into a prediction formula, as follows:

$$X = 5.52 + 0.431Y + 0.552Z,$$

Where X equals the sum of the canine and premolars of one side, Y equals the sum of the four mandibular incisors, and Z equals the mesiodistal width of one mandibular first molar.

The comparative value of the two predictive formulas was tested in a group of randomly selected cases wherein accurate measurments of the sum of the canine and premolars mere available, and it was found that no significant improvement in prediction was afforded by using the more complicated procedure. Accordingly, no further consideration to the use of the mandibular first permanent molars for predictive purposes was given.

The next step was to determine the reliability of the predictive chart, as compared with measurements taken from unerupted teeth in dental x-rays. Sixty determinations were taken as an adequate test.

This was accomplished by measuring from dental x-rays the sum of the mesiodistal widths of unerupted canines, first and second premolars.

↓

In these cases, by using measurements of mandibular incisors taken from mixed dentition models which corresponded in time with the x-rays, the sum of the mesiodistal widths of the mandibular canines and premolars of one side was predicted from the chart shown in Figure.

↓

The accuracy of the measurements from mixed dentition x-rays and of the predicted value was checked by taking divider measurements from models of the same children after eruption of all the permanent teeth.

The films used were intraoral films of average quality and quite comparable with those available to most orthodontists.

The average error in the determination of the sum of these three teeth from x-rays was 10.5 per cent (2.2 millimeters). Although the amount of error varied from one case to another, the error was always in the direction of enlargement. The average error of the predictive graph was 2.6 per cent (0.6 millimeters).

Dr. C. W. Carey of Palo Alto, California, did much to provide the incentive for developing this predictive graph. It was he who measured the mesiodistal widths of permanent teeth in a considerable number of models of his patients, in an effort to arrive at much the same result in cases where dental x-rays proved unsatisfactory. His method was to use an average value for the total mesiodistal width of the canine and premolars of one side when the sum of the four mandibular incisors fell within a certain range.

ADVANTAGES

- This is simple method of estimating the width of the unerupted teeth.
- It is quantitative method of mixed dentition analysis.
- No need for radiographs.

DISADVANTAGES

- Not a substitute for a good set of intraoral films.
- The predictive graph will give only the sum of the unerupted teeth of one side in the mixed dentition, and does not provide an estimate of the mesiodistal width of any one of the three teeth.
- It is offered as an adjunct to the method of the mixed dentition diagnosis and case analysis of Nance.

MORREESS ANALYSIS

This analysis was recommended by COENRAAD F.A. MORREESS, SELMA Ø, THOMSEN, ELLI JENSEN and PETER KAI-JEN YEN in the year 1957. They investigated, by measurements on dental casts of 184 North American children of European ancestry, the relationship between the mesio-distal crown widths of primary and permanent teeth.

Since the crowding and spacing of teeth depend in large measure on the relationship between the size of the bony dental arch and the size of the teeth, the importance of mesiodistal crown diameter as one of the two factors in the equation is clear. The relationship between the mesiodistal crown diameters of the deciduous and permanent teeth likewise plays an important role in the development of occlusion of the permanent dentition. Little information was available concerning this phase of dental development because the longitudinal data needed for its study are difficult to obtain.[11]

AIM

Main purpose of the present study is of an orthodontic nature dealing with the space occupied by the teeth in the dental arch, the findings on mesiodistal crown diameters of single teeth have been combined to obtain the mesiodistal crown diameters of certain groups of teeth.

The relationships between the mesiodistal crown diameters of the deciduous and permanent incisors and canines, as well as those between the deciduous molars and their permanent successors, the premolars, have been determined also by expressing the combined crown diameters of the deciduous teeth as a percentage of that of the permanent teeth.

ARMAMENTARIUM

- Plaster casts
- Modeling compound
- Hydrocolloid material.
- Sliding caliper

PROCEDURE

The material for the present study consisted of plaster casts of the dentitions of 184 North American children of European stock (91 males and 93 females), studied longitudinally from 3 to 18 years of age. Most of these casts (132) were collected as part of the study of "Maternal and Child Health" directed by Dr. Harold C. Stuart of the School of Public Health, Harvard University. The others (52) were gathered by Dr. Richard H. Stucklen in the Bayard Public School in Wilmington, Delaware.

Plaster casts of the dentitions of 184 North American children were obtained

↓

Impressions of the deciduous dentitions were made with modeling compound and those of the permanent dentitions with a hydrocolloid material.

↓

The mesiodistal crown diameter of a tooth was obtained by measuring the greatest distance between the contact points on its proximal surfaces, using a sliding caliper held parallel both to the occlusal and vestibular surfaces.

(When teeth are in normal position)

Otherwise, the mesiodistal crown diameter was obtained by measuring between the points where contact with the neighboring teeth "normally" should occur.

↓

The errors of measurement by different investigators, both of mesiodistal crown diameters of individual permanent teeth and of the combined mesiodistal crown diameters of a series of such teeth (Pm1 - Pm1), were calculated from a number of double determinations and expressed as standard deviations of the differences.

↓

For single permanent mandibular teeth of different tooth classes the error of measurement was 0.09 mm. (n = 360) and for the combined mesiodistal crown diameters of ten permanent mandibular teeth (Pm2 - Pm2) it was 0.41 mm. (n = 30).

For each tooth class statistical analysis of the data on this crown dimension is based on average diameter of the teeth on the right and left side of each dental cast. When, occasionally, the antimere of a tooth is missing, the mesiodistal crown diameter of the one tooth present is used. For these reasons, the "n" values in Tables I and II do not represent the total number of teeth measured, but refer to the number of individuals studied.

TABLE I
MESIODISTAL CROWN DIAMETERS OF DECIDUOUS TEETH OF NORTH AMERICAN WHITE CHILDREN
(MM.)

		M		$S.E._M$	S.D.	RANGE	n	C.R.	p
					Maxilla				
di_1	♂	6.55		0.05	0.36	5.8- 7.2	64	1.56	0.1 $<p<$ 0.15
	♀		6.44	0.05	0.43	5.4- 7.5	69		
di_2	♂	5.32		0.05	0.39	4.5- 6.6	64	1.41	0.15 $<p<$ 0.16
	♀		5.23	0.04	0.33	4.5- 6.2	69		
dc	♂	6.88		0.04	0.36	6.1- 7.9	65	3.63	$p<$ 0.001
	♀		6.67	0.04	0.35	5.9- 7.6	69		
dm_1	♂	7.12		0.05	0.38	6.3- 8.3	64	2.66	0.001 $<p<$ 0.01
	♀		6.95	0.04	0.36	6.3- 7.9	68		
dm_2	♂	9.08		0.06	0.46	8.0-10.4	63	2.61	0.001 $<p<$ 0.01
	♀		8.84	0.07	0.55	7.5-10.0	68		
					Mandible				
di_1	♂	4.08		0.04	0.30	3.0- 4.7	64	1.75	0.05 $<p<$ 0.1
	♀		3.98	0.04	0.30	3.2- 4.7	68		
di_2	♂	4.74		0.04	0.35	4.1- 6.0	65	1.72	0.05 $<p<$ 0.1
	♀		4.63	0.05	0.39	3.9- 5.7	69		
dc	♂	5.92		0.04	0.32	5.1- 6.7	65	3.18	0.001 $<p<$ 0.01
	♀		5.74	0.04	0.35	5.0- 6.6	68		
dm_1	♂	7.80		0.05	0.42	7.0- 8.9	65	2.34	0.01 $<p<$ 0.05
	♀		7.65	0.04	0.35	6.7- 8.5	69		
dm_2	♂	9.83		0.07	0.52	8.5-11.0	63	2.07	0.01 $<p<$ 0.05
	♀		9.64	0.06	0.49	8.6-10.9	69		

TABLE II
MESIODISTAL CROWN DIAMETERS OF PERMANENT TEETH OF NORTH AMERICAN WHITE CHILDREN
(MM.)

		M	$S.E._M$	S.D.	RANGE	n	C.R.	p
				Maxilla				
I_1	♂	8.78	0.05	0.46	7.9-10.0	87	4.87	$p<0.001$
	♀	8.40	0.06	0.53	7.1- 9.8	87		
I_2	♂	6.64	0.07	0.63	4.5- 8.2	84	1.72	$0.05 <p<0.1$
	♀	6.47	0.07	0.62	4.5- 8.5	86		
C	♂	7.95	0.05	0.42	6.6- 9.0	87	6.56	$p<0.001$
	♀	7.53	0.04	0.37	6.9- 8.5	85		
Pm_1	♂	7.01	0.04	0.38	6.1- 8.2	87	2.50	$0.01 <p<0.05$
	♀	6.85	0.05	0.42	5.8- 7.8	84		
Pm_2	♂	6.82	0.04	0.37	5.9- 7.6	86	3.13	$0.001<p<0.01$
	♀	6.62	0.05	0.43	5.2- 7.8	81		
M_1	♂	10.81	0.06	0.56	9.9-12.4	83	3.41	$p<0.001$
	♀	10.52	0.06	0.51	9.4-11.9	85		
M_2	♂	10.35	0.08	0.63	8.5-11.7	65	5.09	$p<0.001$
	♀	9.81	0.07	0.49	8.3-11.8	50		
I_1	♂	5.42	0.03	0.31	4.5- 6.1	85	3.40	$p<0.001$
	♀	5.25	0.04	0.36	4.3- 6.1	87		
I_2	♂	5.95	0.04	0.38	5.2- 6.9	85	2.98	$0.001<p<0.01$
	♀	5.78	0.04	0.38	4.7- 6.8	87		
C	♂	6.96	0.04	0.36	6.2- 8.1	84	8.60	$p<0.001$
	♀	6.47	0.04	0.32	5.8- 7.4	87		
Pm_1	♂	7.07	0.04	0.35	6.4- 8.1	85	3.51	$p<0.001$
	♀	6.87	0.04	0.38	5.9- 7.9	87		
Pm_2	♂	7.29	0.06	0.52	6.3- 9.6	82	3.75	$p<0.001$
	♀	7.02	0.04	0.40	6.2- 7.9	83		
M_1	♂	11.18	0.05	0.47	10.0-12.7	76	5.64	$p<0.001$
	♀	10.74	0.06	0.56	9.4-12.2	84		
M_2	♂	10.76	0.10	0.71	9.3-12.5	53	3.28	$p<0.001$
	♀	10.34	0.08	0.62	9.2-11.7	53		

This procedure was used to obtain the correct standard errors of the means, since the magnitude of a standard error is inversely proportional to the number of observations, i.e., the larger this number, the smaller the error.

By counting the mesiodistal crown diameters for both the right and left teeth of each tooth class separately, the sample no longer consists of completely independent observations, because a tooth and its antimere are influenced by similar, although not necessarily identical, genetic and environmental factors.

For this reason one may be counting the end result of the same factor complex twice in a majority of instances when basing the calculations on the number of individual teeth. The smaller standard error thus obtained may lead to an overestimate of the true level of statistical significance when analyzing the difference between the two means.

RESULTS

The data on mesiodistal crown diameters of the deciduous and permanent maxillary and mandibular teeth of the North American white children studied are summarized in Tables I and II.

- The tooth crowns of the males are seen to be invariably broader than those of the females.

  This sex difference is larger for the permanent than for the deciduous teeth, as indicated by the critical ratios, and it is more pronounced for the canines than for any other teeth in both dentitions.

- The mean mesiodistal crown diameters of the deciduous teeth are smaller for the North American children studied here than for the Swedish children measured by Seipel except in the case of the deciduous maxillary second molars.

  For both sexes these differences are statistically significant, with the exception of those for the deciduous maxillarv central incisors and the maxillarv and mandibular second molars.[10]

- In general, judging from the mean mesiodistal crown diameter obtained, the permanent teeth of the North American children are also smaller.

  Although not always significantly smaller than the teeth in the two samples of Swedish children.

  In the few instances where the opposite relationship seems to exist, the differences found have no statistical significance.

- When comparing the mean mesiodistal crown diameters for the two different samples of Swedish children, statistically significant differences are found for the permanent maxillary and mandibular incisors and canines of the boys and the permanent maxillary and mandibular canines of the girls.

These data are consistent with the usual finding according to which the permanent incisors and canines are larger, but the premolars smaller than their deciduous predecessors. However, a marked range of individual departures from the mean values can be noted from the tabulations. In some instances, the exfoliation of the deciduous molars provides a considerable amount of space in excess of that needed for the emerging premolars, while in other instances; the difference in space requirements is negligible.

A large surplus of space may occur in the maxilla, as well as in the mandible. This happens more often in the mandible than in the maxilla and is made evident by comparing the mean indices expressing the relationship between the mesiodistal crown diameters of the deciduous mandibular molars and the successional premolars in the two jaws.

The combined mesiodistal crown diameters of the maxillary and mandibular deciduous teeth (dm2 - dmi) and of their permanent successors (Pm2 - Pm2) are shown in Table III.

TABLE III
COMBINED MESIODISTAL CROWN DIAMETERS OF THE DECIDUOUS TEETH AND THEIR PERMANENT SUCCESSORS (MM.)

		M		S.E.$_M$	S.D.	RANGE	n	C.R.	p
	Deciduous teeth ($dm_2 - dm_1$)								
Maxilla	♂	69.69		0.37	2.89	63.8-76.9	60	3.17	$0.001 < p < 0.01$
	♀		68.04	0.38	3.04	62.5-76.1	65		
Mandible	♂	64.52		0.37	2.86	59.2-71.9	59	2.57	$p < 0.01$
	♀		63.21	0.35	2.83	56.4-67.4	65		
	Permanent teeth ($Pm_2 - Pm_2$)								
Maxilla	♂	74.91		0.44	3.38	68.4-84.2	57	5.27	$p < 0.001$
	♀		71.63	0.44	3.36	62.4-79.4	57		
Mandible	♂	65.29		0.39	2.93	57.4-72.7	57	4.51	$p < 0.001$
	♀		63.04	0.39	3.11	57.2-70.4	62		

The mean value of these combined crown diameter of the maxillary permanent teeth is 5.22 mm. larger than that of their deciduous predecessors in the males, and 3.59 mm. larger in the females.

In the mandible, the permanent teeth of the males are only 0.77 mm. larger than the deciduous teeth. In the females, on the other hand, the difference between the means is even less, or only 0.17 mm.

The critical ratios of the differences between the mean combined mesiodistal crown diameters in the males and females are again higher for the permanent than for the deciduous dentition, and these differences are statistically significant in all instances (Table III).

The relationship between the mesiodistal crown diameters of the deciduous teeth and their permanent successors has been computed from the formula:

$$\frac{\text{Sum of mesiodistal crown diameters of deciduous teeth } (dm_2 - dm_2)}{\text{Sum of mesiodistal crown diameters of permanent teeth } (Pm_2 - Pm_2)} \times 100.$$

The mean figure expressing the sum of the mesiodistal crown diameters of the deciduous teeth in terms of a percentage of that of the corresponding permanent teeth is 93 for the maxillary dentition of the males and 95 for the females; in the mandibular dentition the corresponding percentages are 98 and 100, respectively. These findings support the conclusions previously made from the absolute measurements (Table III).

ADVANTAGES

- There is the possibility of calculating the correlation coefficient or the degree of association between the mesiodistal crown diameters of the deciduous and permanent teeth in the same subject.
- No need of radiographs.

Although differing significantly from zero, except for the maxillary lateral incisors in males, the degree of association between the mesiodistal crown diameters of the deciduous and permanent teeth of each tooth class was found to be low to medium with coefficients ranging from +0.23 to +0.65 (Table IV).

TABLE IV
CORRELATION COEFFICIENTS FOR MESIODISTAL CROWN DIAMETERS OF CORRESPONDING SINGLE AND COMBINED DECIDUOUS AND PERMANENT TEETH

	MALES			FEMALES		
	r	S.E.$_r$	n	r	S.E.$_r$	n
Maxilla						
$di_1 : I_1$	+0.56	±0.09	64	+0.65	±0.07	66
$di_2 : I_2$	+0.23*	±0.12	61	+0.41	±0.10	65
dc : C	+0.26	±0.12	64	+0.34	±0.11	64
$dm_1 : Pm_1$	+0.27	±0.12	63	+0.34	±0.11	62
$dm_2 : Pm_2$	+0.34	±0.11	62	+0.45	±0.10	59
$dm_2 - dm_2 : Pm_2 - Pm_2$	+0.54	±0.10	56	+0.69	±0.07	57
Mandible						
$di_1 : I_1$	+0.43	±0.10	62	+0.37	±0.11	65
$di_2 : I_2$	+0.35	±0.11	63	+0.39	±0.10	66
dc : C	+0.28	±0.12	63	+0.32	±0.11	65
$dm_1 : Pm_1$	+0.41	±0.11	63	+0.53	±0.09	64
$dm_2 : Pm_2$	+0.37	±0.11	58	+0.42	±0.10	64
$dm_2 - dm_2 : Pm_2 - Pm_2$	+0.59	±0.09	55	+0.49	±0.10	61

*The correlation coefficient does not differ significantly from zero.

Thus, in general, deciduous teeth with a small mesiodistal crown diameter are succeeded by permanent teeth which are likewise small in their mesiodistal dimension, while broad deciduous teeth are likely to be followed by broad permanent ones.

Yet, the relatively low numerical values of the correlation coefficients indicate that in individual instances a great deal of variation can be expected in the size of permanent tooth replacing a deciduous tooth of a given mesiodistal crown diameter.

The highest correlation coefficient was found for the mesiodistal crown diameters of the deciduous and permanent maxillary central incisors (r = +0.56 for males and 40.65 for females). It is obvious, then, that no accurate prediction of the mesiodistal crown diameter of the permanent tooth can be made even in this particular instance, on the basis of a measurement of its deciduous predecessor.

CONCLUSION

The correlation coefficient was low, reflecting great individual variation within the population. A sex difference was noted, males having larger teeth than females; therefore the results were analysed for males and females separately. He found that permanent incisor and canine teeth were larger than their predecessors, whereas premolar teeth were smaller. He concluded that measurement of unerupted permanent canines and premolars on radiographs was more accurate than estimation by measurement of the primary dentition.

TANAKA AND JOHNSTON ANALYSIS

This is a non radiographic method of mixed dentition analysis suggested by MARVIN M. TANAKA and LYSLE E. JOHNSTON of Cleveland in 1974. They developed probability equation to predict mesiodistal width of unerupted canine and premolars by using sum of four mandibular incisors.[5]

Dental casts for 506 orthodontic patients in the Cleveland area were obtained from the orthodontic department of Case Western Reserve University School of Dentistry and from the records of three orthodontists practicing in the Cleveland area, Drs. Sanford Neuger, Arthur Phelps, and Milton Rabine.

- The Tanaka and Johnston method of arch-length analysis is a variation of Moyers' analysis except that a prediction table is not needed.

- It is recomandable as a predictive technique because it has reasonable accuracy, does not require radiographs, requires no prediction tables and predicts the sizes of the unerupted permanent canines and premolars in maxillary and mandibular teeth.[25]

INCLUSION CRITERIA

- Patients had to be of probable European ancestry and less than 20 years old.
- Teeth to be measured had to be fully erupted.
- Free of visible fractures, caries, and restorations.

ARMAMENTARIUM

- Dental casts

- Pointed vernier calipers
- Programmable electronic calculator

PROCEDURE

- Mesiodistal widths of the permanent mandibular incisors and all canines and premolars were obtained with pointed vernier calipers, and they were read to the nearest 0.05 mm according to methods outlined by Seipel and Moorrees. [10,11]
- The moderately high degree of linear correlation that exists among various groups of permanent teeth makes it possible to measure the total width of the permanent mandibular incisors and to predict the size of teeth that have yet to erupt.
- The data was used to generate formulas—"regression" equations—that can be used clinically to effect predictions in much the same way one converts Farenheit to Celsius.
- Specifically, least-squares regression equations of the form Y=A+B (X) were calculated with a programmable electronic calculator. In these equations,
    - Y equals the predicted size of an unerupted buccal segment (canine and premolars);
    - X equals the measured width of the four mandibular incisors;
    - A and B are constants.

Coefficients of linear correlation, standard errors of estimate, and confidence belts for individual predictions were calculated for each equation in the evaluation of the accuracy of the resulting formulas.

According to Dean et al, the estimated width in millimeters, of unerupted canines and premolars measured with Tanaka and Johnston method corresponded to the 75% level of probability in Moyer's prediction table.

Used the following measurements

1. Half the mesiodistal width of 4 lower incisor + 10.5 = mandibular 3+4+5 in one quadrant.
2. Half the mesiodistal width of 4 lower incisors + 11.0 = Maxillary 3+4+5 in one quadrant.

RESULTS

- Descriptive statistics for the three groups of teeth measured here are presented (Table1).

Table 1 ▪ Descriptive statistics for combined mesiodistal widths in millimeters.

Tooth group	Range	Mean	Standard deviation
Mandibular lateral & central incisors	18.5 to 28.0	23.43	1.35
Maxillary canines, first premolars, & second premolars	19.1 to 25.9	22.27	1.09
Mandibular canines, first premolars, & second premolars	18.4 to 24.9	21.76	1.12

- Coefficients of correlation for the canine-premolar segments of each dental arch, and the values of A, B, and the standard errors of estimate for the two regression equations are shown (Table 2).

Table 2 ▪ Prediction equations.

Canine-premolar segment	Coefficient of correlation	Regression coefficients		Standard error of estimate in millimeters
		A	B	
Maxillary	0.625	10.41	0.51	0.86
Mandibular	0.648	9.18	0.54	0.85

- Percentiles for the prediction of the size of maxillary and mandibular buccal segments are presented in (Tables 3 and 4) respectively.

Table 3 ▪ Probability table for predicting the widths of maxillary canines, first premolars, and second premolars from mandibular lateral and central incisors in millimeters.

	Mandibular lateral and central incisors													
	20.5	21.0	21.5	22.0	22.5	23.0	23.5	24.0	24.5	25.0	25.5	26.0	26.5	27.0
95%	22.2	22.5	22.7	23.0	23.2	23.5	23.7	24.0	24.2	24.5	24.7	25.0	25.2	25.5
85%	21.7	21.9	22.2	22.4	22.7	22.9	23.2	23.4	23.7	24.0	24.2	24.5	24.7	25.0
75%	21.4	21.6	21.9	22.1	22.4	22.6	22.9	23.1	23.4	23.6	23.9	24.1	24.4	24.7
65%	21.1	21.4	21.6	21.9	22.1	22.4	22.6	22.9	23.1	23.4	23.6	23.9	24.2	24.4
50%	20.8	21.0	21.3	21.5	21.8	22.1	22.3	22.6	22.8	23.1	23.3	23.6	23.8	24.1
35%	20.5	20.7	21.0	21.2	21.5	21.7	22.0	22.2	22.5	22.7	23.0	23.2	23.5	23.7
25%	20.2	20.5	20.7	21.0	21.2	21.5	21.7	22.0	22.2	22.5	22.7	23.0	23.2	23.5
15%	19.9	20.1	20.4	20.7	20.9	21.2	21.4	21.7	21.9	22.2	22.4	22.7	22.9	23.2
5%	19.4	19.6	19.9	20.1	20.4	20.6	20.9	21.1	21.4	21.7	21.9	22.2	22.4	22.7

Table 4 ▪ Probability table for predicting the widths of mandibular canines, first premolars, and second premolars from mandibular lateral and central incisors in millimeters.

	Mandibular lateral and central incisors													
	20.5	21.0	21.5	22.0	22.5	23.0	23.5	24.0	24.5	25.0	25.5	26.0	26.5	27.0
95%	21.6	21.9	22.1	22.4	22.7	22.9	23.2	23.5	23.7	24.0	24.3	24.5	24.8	25.1
85%	21.1	21.3	21.6	21.9	22.1	22.4	22.7	23.0	23.2	23.5	23.8	24.0	24.3	24.6
75%	20.8	21.0	21.3	21.6	21.8	22.1	22.3	22.6	22.9	23.2	23.4	23.7	24.0	24.3
65%	20.5	20.8	21.1	21.3	21.6	21.9	22.1	22.4	22.7	22.9	23.2	23.5	23.7	24.0
50%	20.2	20.5	20.7	21.0	21.3	21.5	21.8	22.1	22.3	22.6	22.9	23.1	23.4	23.7
35%	19.9	20.1	20.4	20.7	20.9	21.2	21.5	21.7	22.0	22.3	22.5	22.8	23.1	23.3
25%	19.6	19.9	20.1	20.4	20.7	21.0	21.2	21.5	21.8	22.0	22.3	22.6	22.8	23.1
15%	19.3	19.6	19.8	20.1	20.4	20.6	20.9	21.2	21.5	21.7	22.0	22.3	22.5	22.8
5%	18.8	19.0	19.3	19.6	19.9	20.1	20.4	20.7	20.9	21.2	21.5	21.7	22.0	22.3

- The regression coefficients that were remarkably similar to those of Ballard and Wylie (mandible, A=9.41 and B=0.527) and Moyers (by inference: maxilla, A=9.23 and B=0.55; mandible, A=7.82 and B=0.60). Indeed, all statistics were so similar that confidence belts match Moyers's almost exactly (Table 5).

Table 5 ▪ Comparison of probability tables for canines, first premolars, and second premolars: the 75th percentile.

Width of mandibular incisors (mm)	Width of maxillary canines, first premolars, and second premolars (mm)			Width of mandibular canines, first premolars, and second premolars (mm)		
	Moyers	CWRU*	Approximation	Moyers	CWRU*	Approximation
20.5	21.2	21.4	21.3	20.7	20.8	20.8
21.0	21.5	21.6	21.5	21.0	21.0	21.0
21.5	21.8	21.9	21.8	21.3	21.3	21.3
22.0	22.0	22.1	22.0	21.6	21.6	21.5
22.5	22.3	22.4	22.3	21.9	21.8	21.8
23.0	22.6	22.6	22.5	22.2	22.1	22.0
23.5	22.9	22.9	22.8	22.5	22.3	22.3
24.0	23.1	23.1	23.0	22.8	22.6	22.5
24.5	23.4	23.4	23.3	23.1	22.9	22.8
25.0	23.7	23.6	23.5	23.4	23.2	23.0
25.5	24.0	23.9	23.8	23.7	23.4	23.3
26.0	24.2	24.1	24.0	24.0	23.7	23.5
26.5	24.5	24.4	24.3	24.3	24.0	23.8
27.0	24.8	24.7	24.5	24.6	24.3	24.0

ADVANTAGES:

- Simple, easy and relatively non invasive and accurate.
- Applicable for both dental arches and genders.[37]
- Significant clinical acceptability.
- Minimal amount of time and effort.
- Regression equations for the combined black males and females were found to be in close agreement with Tanaka's regression equations for the maxillary and mandibular arches.[19]

DRAWBACKS:

- Tanaka and Johnston method does not takes into account the axial inclination of mandibular anterior teeth, the effects of curve of spee, inner prediction bias, ethnic group biases or facial profile, all of which can affect the amount of crowding and space required in analysis.[25]

- Analysis are based on populations of other racial origin, hence the prediction must be done with care.

- The findings indicated that on the average the Tanaka and Johnston approach slightly overestimated the tooth size of the unerupted teeth.[3]

Studies on validation of Tanaka and Johnston's analysis to different population:

Using simple linear regression analyses, prediction equations for the combined mesiodistal crown diameters of canines and premolars based on lower incisor size were generated from 97 Hong Kong Chinese (51 males and 46 females, average age 12.31 years) out of a sample of 112. The mesiodistal crown diameters of the permanent teeth were measured using calipers and recorded to the nearest 0.01 mm. Significant sex differences were found for the combined diameters of the canine-premolar segments. The coefficients of correlation between combined diameters of canines and premolars and lower incisors ranged from 0.65 to 0.79. Significant sex differences of the regression equations were found and thus four simple linear regression equations were generated. Coefficients for the slope ranged from 0.58 to 0.66, and coefficients for the intercept ranged from 6.66 to 8.82. The R2 values, standard errors of estimate, and absolute mean errors revealed that prediction models for females were less precise than those for males. Probability tables were constructed from the results of the present study. The prediction equations were found to differ from those of Tanaka and Johnston. Accuracy in the mixed dentition analysis for southern Chinese would be improved by applying the prediction equations or probability tables generated from the present study.[66]

In the study undertaken by Sharon Lee Chan et al in 1998, 201 dental plaster casts of Asia-Pacific-American subjects, all of whom were under the age of 21 years, were used. The actual measurements were compared with the predicted values derived from the Tanaka and Johnston equations and significant differences were found. The data illustrate the limitations of the Tanaka and Johnston method when applied to a sample population of other than European descent. From this data, two linear regression equations were developed for tooth size prediction in Asian-American children.[66]

Maxillary: Y = 8.2 + 0.6 (X)

Mandibular: Y = 7.5 + 0.6 (X)

X = Mesiodistal width of the four mandibular incisors in millimeters.

Y = Mesiodistal width of the canine and premolars in one quadrant in millimeters.

With the aim to validate Tanaka and Johnston's analysis on 600 Syrian patients aged 14–22 years a study was undertaken by Nourallah et al in 2002. Tanaka and Johnston's tables, equations, and approximations were modified in order to improve the accuracy of the prediction. The correlation coefficients found between the size of the permanent mandibular central incisors and maxillary first molars (31, 41, 16, and 26) and the maxillary and mandibular canines and premolars were high ($r = .72$ and .74, respectively). New, more accurate prediction tables applicable at earlier ages, and new regression equations were constructed. In addition, new easier approximations were developed to allow the prediction of the size of the unerupted maxillary canines and premolars by adding 6 mm to the half-widths of teeth 31, 41, 16, and 26. The analogous prediction of the size of the unerupted mandibular canines and premolars was obtained by adding 5.5 mm to the half-widths of same teeth, 31, 41, 16, and 26. [27]

Study was undertaken by E.R. Altherr et al in 2007 to determine the predictive accuracy of the Tanaka-Johnston analysis in white and black subjects in North Carolina .The predicted widths of the canines and the premolars in both arches were compared with the actual measured widths.In the maxillary arch, there was a significant interaction of ethnicity and sex on the predictive accuracy of the Tanaka-Johnston analysis ($P = .03$). The predictive accuracy was significantly overestimated in the white female group ($P < .001$, least square means). In the mandibular arch, there was no significant interaction between ethnicity and sex ($P = .49$) and underestimated in blacks ($P < .0001$) (factorial ANOVA). Regression equations were developed to increase the predictive accuracy in both arches.[67]

Regression equations are widely used for mixed dentition analysis. However, estimations from these equations can vary in different population groups. This study was conducted to produce simple linear equations and tables for Pakistani children. Two hundred subjects of Pakistani descent who met our criteria (ages, 13-15 years; 100 boys, 100 girls) were selected from local schools. The mesiodistal widths of all mandibular permanent incisors, canines, and premolars were measured and analyzed. The results were also compared with predicted values from the Moyers and the Tanaka and Johnston methods. Correlation and linear regression analyses were performed between the predicted and actual tooth sizes for Pakistani children and standard regression equations were developed. No significant differences were observed for measured canine and premolar antimeres and sex. Significant and high positive correlations were found between the mandibular incisors and the combined mesiodistal widths of the canines and premolarsfor the maxillary (r 5 0.65; P\0.001) and mandibular (r 5 0.59; P\0.001) segments. Conclusions: The equations and charts commonly used for North American children (75th percentile) did not accurately predict for their sample. The regression equations and tables developed in this study can be used for orthodontic treatment planning for children in Pakistan.[36]

A study was conducted to determine the modified equations from Tanaka and Johnston for Iranian population. This study was an analytic and cross-sectional investigation with the randomized cluster sampling in Ahwaz. Fifty four students of 14-18 years age (32 girls, 22 boys) were selected between 320 students and plaster models of their maxillary and mandibular arches were prepared. Subjects had fully erupted teeth, class I canine and molar relationship and presented no proximal caries or fillings, morphological anomalies, missing teeth or occlusal abrasion, and bruxism. The mesiodistal crown diameters of the permanent teeth were measured with using the sharpened boley gauge (accuracy 0.01 mm). The data were analyzed by using the regression correlation analyses. The size of permanent canines and premolars were larger in maxilla than mandible and males than females. These values in Iran were different from other countries. In this study to predict the space (in mm) required for alignment of unerupted canine and premolars in Iranian children, halve the sum of mesiodistal dimension of the four mandibular incisors and add the respective constants 10.5 for upper jaw and 10 for lower jaw.[38]

A study was carried out to determine the correlation between the sum of the mandibular permanent incisors and the combined mesiodistal crown diameters of the maxillary and mandibular canine and premolars in a sample of mixed Indian subjects, examine the applicability of the Tanaka and Johnston method of prediction in a mixed Indian population and develop a new prediction method for this specific population. The dental models of the dentition of 251 mixed Indian patients below the age of 21 years, who had upper and lower permanent canines and premolars erupted were selected for this study. All the measurements were made with modified Boley gauge with Vernier caliper. The differences between the predicted widths of the canine and premolars with the Tanaka and Johnston equations and the actual widths were highly statistically significant. The actual widths of the maxillary canine and premolars showed a significant difference in size from the widths predicted by the Tanaka and Johnston equation, as did the canine and premolars in the mandible. The findings suggest that the accuracy of originally derived Tanaka and Johnston mixed dentition analysis method can be increased using a newly derived regression equations based on a local mixed Indian population.[45]

MOYER'S ANALYSIS (1963):-

The Moyers analysis based on measurements of erupted teeth is one of the techniques that enjoys wide clinical acceptance due to its relative ease of application and interpretation

- It is a non radiographic method of mixed dentition space analysis.
- Moyer's method is more widely used mixed dentition space analysis.[34]
- Moyer suggested two probability tables to predict the sizes of unerupted teeth in mixed dentition using the sum of the widths of four mandibular permanent incisiors.
- Mandibular incisors are been chosen for measuring, since they erupt early in mixed dentition period.
- The maxillary incisiors show too much variability in size and their correlations with other groups of teeth are of lower predictive value and so not chosen.
- The range and variability in predictions were always smaller with the Moyers technique compared to simple visual observation (SVO).[28]

.

PROCEDURE IN MANDIBULAR ARCH:-

- With the help of Boley's gauge measure the mesio- distal width of each of the four mandibular incisors.

↓

- To determine the amount of space required for the alignment of incisors, set the guage to the value of the sum of central and lateral incisor of one side.

↓

- Place one point of Boley's guage at the midline and let the other end lie along the dental arch on the side of the central and lateral incisors whose widths were measured. Mark this point on the cast. It represents the point at which the distal surface of the lateral incisor will be when it has been aligned properly. Repeat this for the opposite side.

↓

- To determine the amount of space available for the permanent canine and premolars after incisor alignment measure the distance from the point marked on the cast to the mesial surface of first permanent molar.

↓

- The combined width of the mandibular canines and premolars is then predicted with the help of the probability chart. The value corresponding to the sum of the widths of the mandibular incisors is located at the top of the chart. The range of values for canines and premolars can be recorded.

↓

- The estimated canine and premolar size value is subtracted from the measured space. It is assumed that the molar will move usually by 1.7mm on each side. After

↓

recording the values, complete assessment of the space in both the arches is possible.

- The value at the 75% level of probability is chosen as the estimate, since it has been found to be the most practical from a clinical stand point.

PROCEDURE IN MAXILLARY ARCH:-

- A different probability chart is used for predicting the sum of upper cuspid and bicuspid.

↓

- Allowance must be made for overjet correction when measuring the space to be occupied by aligned incisors.

↓

- The width of the lower incisors is use to predict upper cuspid and bicuspid widths.

ADVANTAGES

1. Minimal known systematic error.
2. Can be used by beginner and expert with equal reliability.
3. Less time consuming.
4. Doesn't require specific equipment or exposure to radiographs.
5. Applicable to both upper and lower dental arches.

6. Best done on dental cast bit it can be done in mouth with reasonable accuracy
7. The basis for this analysis is the tooth size. (i.e.) on measuring the size of a tooth or a group of teeth the size of other teeth can be predicted.

DISADVANTAGES

1. Although Moyer's method has advantages, it was developed on a Caucasian population. The applicability of this method to populations of other ethnic groups has been studied and doubted.
2. It requires a special chart for prediction of width of canine and premolars.

- Zilberman, Koyoumdjisk-Kaye, and Vardimon checked the accuracy of the Moyersand Hixon-Oldfather estimations in a group of forty-six Israeli children. They found a stronger correlation in both arches between observed sizes and measurements from the x-ray films than from the Moyers' tables. The scatter around the regression line based on Moyers' estimate was larger than that around the regression line based on x-ray finding.[16]
- The percentage of overestimation was more for Tanaka – Johnston prediction method than that of Moyers (75th percentile).[43]
- The analysis allowed for the space required for tooth alignment and retroclination of the labial segment, if necessary.[8]

Studies on applicability and validation of Moyers MDA in different population

The mixed dentition analysis described by Moyers, and later validated by Tanaka, was performed on 80 American blacks to compare prediction equations between Caucasians and blacks. For the black sample, separate regression formulas were determined for the 39 males and 41 females and the combined black sample. Although sexual dimorphism of tooth size was not a consideration in the Moyers prediction charts, this research evaluated the effect of sexual dimorphism in the mixed dentition analysis. Regression equations were generated by the method of least squares, and the 2-tailed t-test was used to determine significant differences between 2 equations for the same arch. The findings include a significant difference for the mandibular regression equation for black males when compared with (1) the Tanaka equation for Caucasians and (2) the regression equation for black females. Maxillary regression equations were not significantly different between the Caucasian and black samples or between black males and females.[19]

Hakason compared data obtained using the Moyers probability chart for a sample of Caucasian, Negro and oriental children. He found the Moyers analysis to underestimate the total required size of the permanent canine and premolars in the maxilla and mandible for the three racial groups and suggested that an adjustment be made in using the Moyers predictability table for Negro and oriental children where by 0.7 mm would be added to the total mesio-distal diameter of the maxillary permanent canine and premolar size estimates. In the mandibular arch, 1.20 mm should be added to measurements for Negro children estimates only. In this case the oriental and Caucasian measurements coincide with those on the Moyer's chart.

Data were collected from a series of 100 randomly selected study models of black patients. The sample was equally subdivided by gender and all subjects had Angle Class I molar relationships with only minor malocclusions such as minor crowding, rotations, or diastemas. Intra-examiner and inter-examiner reliability was determined at 0.2 mm. All teeth to and including the first molars were measured. These data were then utilized in regression equations for both maxillary and mandibular arches, to enable the prediction of the mesiodistal widths of the canines and two premolars. The equations and predicted values were compared with those of the Moyers' probability tables, and significant differences ($p<0.05$) were found (except for the prediction of maxillary canines and premolars in females at the 85 and 95percentile probability level). New probability tables for black subjects were formulated. It is envisaged that the proposed probability tables would be more accurate for black patients of African ancestry.[23]

A meta-analysis to assess the applicability of Moyer's method in different ethnic groups, done by William Buwembo et al included seven articles in the study by a literature search of Medline (1966–June 2003). 195 articles were reviewed and meta-analyzed. Separation of the articles into Caucasian and Asian groups gave borderline p-values of 0.05. Variation in the correlation coefficients of different populations using Moyer's method may fall either side. This implies that Moyer's method of prediction may have population variations. For one to be sure of the accuracy while using Moyer's method it may be safer to develop prediction tables for specific populations. Thus Moyer's method cannot universally be applied without question.[29]

Sushma sonawane et al did a study on Marathi population in 2008 for applicability of Moyer's mixed dentition analysis. It was concluded that using Moyers analysis at 50% confidence level, gives a realistic values. The regression equation obtained for mandibular and maxillary teeth were:

For mandibular teeth, Y = 10.830 + 0.563 (X)

For maxillary teeth, Y = 12.143 + 0.481 (X) [68]

Study done by Sujala Ganapati Durgekar et al in 2008 to test the reliability of Moyers mixed dentition analysis in school children in Belgaum, Karnataka, India in 150 school children within the age group of 13 to 16 years old who had all permanent teeth were included. Mesiodistal dimensions of permanent mandibular incisors, maxillary and mandibular canines, and premolars were measured using a digital caliper with a resolution of 0.01 mm. The actual measurements were compared with the predicted values obtained with the Moyers prediction tables at the 35th, 50th, and 75th percentile confidence levels. Using this data, linear regression equations were formulated for tooth size prediction. The coefficient of determination [r2] was calculated to find the accuracy of the formulated prediction equations. The standard error of estimate (SEE) was calculated to determine the validity of the proposed equations. Moyers prediction tables are not an accurate method to estimate tooth dimension in our samples. The mesiodistal crown dimension in the buccal segment of the mandibular arch was larger in males (p=0.04) than in females. They concluded that the differences between predicted values from the Moyers tables and that of the present investigation are the result of racial and ethnic diversity. The accuracy of the prediction equation should be tested in a larger sample.[32]

Odontometric data were collected by N. I. Phillip et al in 2010 from 300 male and 300 female subjects of Indian descent, who had fully erupted mandibular permanent incisors and maxillary and mandibular canines and premolars. We measured the mesiodistal crown widths with Vernier calipers. All tooth groups showed significant differences (P\0.001) between mesiodistal widths of male and female subjects. Regression equations for the maxillary arch (males, Y = 7.15 + 0.67X; females, Y = 7.44 + 0.65X) and the mandibular arch (males, Y = 5.55 + 0.71X; females, Y = 6.15 + 0.67X) were used to develop new probability tables on the Moyers pattern. Significant differences (P \0.05) were found between our predicted widths and the Moyers tables at almost all percentile levels, including the recommended 75% and 50% levels. These new prediction aids could be considered for a more precise mixed dentition space analysis in Indian children.[35]

A study was undertaken by Shah and Bhaskar in 2013 with the aim to evaluate the accuracy of Melgaço's method in comparison with Moyers' mixed dentition analysis table in contemporary Indian population. Sixty boys and 60 girls from Gandhinagar district (age ranged from 12 to 14 years) were included. The mesiodistal crown widths of all fully erupted teeth were measured with digital verniercallipers and the odontometric values obtained were then subjected to statistical and linear regression analysis. Student's unpaired *t*-test gave statistically significant difference between the original values of teeth and the values obtained by Melgaço's prediction equation as well as Moyers' mixed dentition analysis table ($P < 0.001$). High values of correlation ($r = 0.77$)

and determination coefficients ($r^2 = 0.59$) were found while considering Melgaço's method. Also, no statistically significant difference was found between the tooth sizes of males and females. It can be evaluated that Melgaço's method gives better prediction and a simplified equation $Y = 0.925X$ can be suggested for the present population. [40]

A systematic review was conducted by Galvao et al in 2013, computerized search involving articles published on PubMed and Lilacs between 1990 and September, 2011 in accordance with the method described in the Cochrane 5.1.0 handbook.The research resulted in a sample composed of 629 articles. The inclusion criteria were Articles using the Moyers analysis with a sample greater or equal to 40 patients. For this systematic review, 19 articles were selected. Based on the literature available, it was concluded that the Moyers mixed dentition analysis must be carefully used, since the majority of the articles analyzed showed that the probability of 75% was not as accurate as expected, leading to the need of adapting the probability levels depending on the study population.[39]

The study was aimed to determine the applicability of Moyers mixed dentition arch analysis in children of Baddi, Himachal Pradesh. Dental study models of 120 children in age group of 13- 16 years, were analysed who presented with complete eruption of permanent mandibular incisors, maxillary and mandibular canines & premolars. Measurements of the mesiodistal dimensions of the mandibular and maxillary teeth were made using a digital caliper with a Vernier scale that was calibrated to the nearest 0.01mm. All tooth groups showed highly significant differences ($p<0.001$) between mesiodistal widths in male and female subjects. Significant differences ($p<0.05$) were found between actual widths and the Moyers tables at almost all percentile levels, including the recommended 75%. The differences noted might be the result of racial and ethnic diversity.[41]

Themmegowda et al in 2015 collected data from study models of 400 randomly selected Bangalore subjects aged 13 to 16 years with fully erupted, intact dentitions and no significant malocclusion. The mesiodistal widths of the incisors, canines and premolars of both arches were measured. This data was then utilized to predict the mesiodistal widths of canines and premolars and further compared with Moyer's table.It was found that 50% is more applicable to boys and 75% to girls. The canine premolar segment in both arches is statistically larger in men than in women ($p<0.05$). New regression equation was formulated, the accuracy of which needs to be evaluated further in a larger sample.[44]

The study was undertaken to evaluate the applicability of Moyers' mixed dentition analysis to Bengali and Keralite population, to assess the percentage probability to be used for the two populations Bengali and Keralite. Record casts of 100 Bengali (50 - Males; 50 - Females) of 12-14 years were selected, and mesiodistal width of permanent incisors, canines, premolars was measured on study models. Similarly, 100 samples were drawn from Keralite population. Study models of 50 males and 50 females were prepared, and measurements were made. Paired t-test of difference between actual and predicted values for Bengali samples were least in case of the 65th percentile of the level of significance in upper arch and in lower arch it was the 50th percentile level of significance. For females, mean difference of upper arch was least at 65th percentile level and for lower arch at 50th percentile level of significance. For Keralite population, it was at 50th percentile level of significance in upper and lower arch for male and female it was at 65th percentile level in upper arch and 50th percentile level in the lower arch. The predicted value and the actual value were significantly correlated and may be used with much confidence in estimating the width of permanent canine, first premolar, and second premolar. Moyers' prediction values at 75th percentile level over predicted width of canine and premolars. Moyers prediction values at 65th percentile level of significance may be accepted for predicting the combined width of canine and first and second premolars in case of upper for Bengali male and female and also for upper teeth in Keralite females. In the case of lower arch, values should be accepted at 50th percentile level of significance to get a more accurate prediction.[46]

Prediction table for maxillary arch in males with Moyer's probability chart

L*	75th percentile	50th percentile	35th percentile	Present 75th
19.5	20.3	19.7	19.3	19.84
20.0	20.5	19.9	19.6	20.14
20.5	20.8	20.2	19.9	20.52
21.0	21.0	20.4	20.1	20.62
21.5	21.3	20.7	20.4	20.86
22.0	21.5	20.9	20.6	21.02
22.5	21.8	21.2	20.9	21.35
23.0	22.0	21.5	21.1	21.61
23.5	22.3	21.7	21.4	21.82
24.0	22.5	22.0	21.6	22.15
24.5	22.8	22.2	21.9	22.34
25.0	23.0	22.5	22.1	22.61
25.5	23.3	22.7	22.4	22.78

L=Sum of mandibular incisors*

Prediction chart for mandibular arch in males with Moyer's probability chart

L*	75th percentile	50th percentile	35th percentile	Present 75th
19.5	20.4	19.5	19.0	19.31
20.0	20.6	19.7	19.3	19.42
20.5	20.8	20.0	19.5	19.68
21.0	21.0	20.2	19.7	19.86
21.5	21.2	20.4	20.0	20.18
22.0	21.4	20.6	20.2	20.45
22.5	21.6	20.9	20.4	20.72
23.0	21.9	21.1	20.6	20.92
23.5	22.1	21.3	20.9	21.15
24.0	22.3	21.5	21.1	21.46
24.5	22.5	21.7	21.3	21.83
25.0	22.8	22.0	21.5	21.97
25.5	23.0	22.2	21.7	22.18

L=Sum of mandibular incisors*

Prediction table for maxillary arch in females with Moyer's probability chart

L*	75th percentile	50th percentile	35th percentile	Present 75th
19.5	20.4	19.6	19.2	19.75
20.0	20.5	19.8	19.4	19.92
20.5	20.6	19.9	19.5	20.21
21.0	20.8	20.1	19.7	20.46
21.5	20.9	20.2	19.8	20.59
22.0	21.0	20.3	19.9	20.81
22.5	21.2	20.5	20.1	20.97
23.0	21.3	20.6	20.2	21.15
23.5	21.5	20.8	20.4	21.34
24.0	21.6	20.9	20.5	21.54
24.5	21.8	21.0	20.6	21.74
25.0	21.9	21.2	20.8	21.95
25.5	22.1	21.3	20.9	22.21

L=Sum of mandibular incisors*

Prediction chart for mandibular arch in females with Moyer's probability chart

L*	75th percentile	50th percentile	35th percentile	Present 75th
19.5	19.6	18.7	18.2	19.17
20.0	19.8	19.0	18.5	19.38
20.5	20.1	19.2	18.8	19.61
21.0	20.3	19.5	19.0	19.82
21.5	20.6	19.8	19.3	20.15
22.0	20.8	20.0	19.6	20.28
22.5	21.1	20.3	19.8	20.41
23.0	21.3	20.5	20.1	20.68
23.5	21.6	20.8	20.3	20.91
24.0	21.9	21.1	20.6	21.06
24.5	22.1	21.3	20.9	21.31
25.0	22.4	21.6	21.1	21.46
25.5	22.7	21.8	21.4	21.71

L=Sum of mandibular incisors*

CONCLUSION

The prudent clinician should carefully perform the measurements required for an arch length analysis and use the information thus gained, together with other observations taken from the patient records, to arrive at a decision based on his or her best judgment for each patient. One must remember that in addition to tooth size, the changes in arch dimensions as well as tooth position and inclination are, in part, compensatory mechanisms that maintain the balance among the various functional and structural demands placed on the face and dentition. Many of these changes are difficult to predict in the deciduous dentition stage.

Clinicians and researchers are interested in predicting the potential for a tooth size-arch length discrepancy in their growing patients. If accurate predictions can be made while patients are in the deciduous or mixed dentition, clinicians might attempt to intercept any developing malocclusions. On the other hand, if such discrepancies cannot be accurately predicted, one will have to question the advisability of such procedures.

The most accurate predictons of the mesio-distal widths of unerupted canines and premolars can be obtained by measurements of mesio-distal widths of these teeth on radiographs combined with measurement of mesio-distal widths of the erupted mandibular permanent teeth.

BIBLIOGRAPHY

1. William R. Proffit: Williams R. Proffit, Henry W. Fields, and David M. Sarver's *Contemporary Orthodontics – Fifth Edition*, published by Elsevier.
2. Huckaba GW. Arch size analysis and tooth size prediction. Dental Clinics of North Americqa 1964; 11: 431-40
3. Bishara SE, Jakobsen JR. Comparison of two nonradiographic methods of predicting permanent tooth size in the mixed dentition. American journal of orthodontics and dentofacial orthopedics. 1998 Nov 1;114(5):573-6.
4. Nance HN. The limitations of orthodontic treatment: I. Mixed dentition diagnosis and treatment. American Journal of Orthodontics and Oral Surgery. 1947 Apr 1;33(4):177-223.
5. Tanaka MM, Johnston LE. The prediction of the size of unerupted canines and premolars in a contemporary orthodontic population. The Journal of the American Dental Association. 1974 Apr 1;88(4):798-801.
6. Hixon EH, Oldfather RE. Estimation of the sizes of unerupted cuspid and bicuspid teeth. The Angle Orthodontist. 1958 Oct;28(4):236-40.
7. Foster HR, Wylie WL. Arch length deficiency in the mixed dentition. American Journal of Orthodontics and Dentofacial Orthopedics. 1958 Jun 1;44(6):464-76.
8. Irwin RD, Herold JS, Richardson A. Mixed dentition analysis: a review of methods and their accuracy. International journal of paediatric dentistry. 1995 Sep;5(3):137-42.

9. Ballard ML, Wylie WL. Mixed dentition case analysis-estimating size of unerupted permanent teeth. American Journal of Orthodontics and Dentofacial Orthopedics. 1947 Nov 1;33(11):754-9.
10. Seipel CM. Variations of tooth position: a metric study of variation and adaptation in the deciduous and permanent dentition. American Journal of Orthodontics and Dentofacial Orthopedics. 1948;34:369-72.
11. Moorrees CF, Thomsen SØ, Jensen E, Yen PK. Mesiodistal crown diameters of the deciduous and permanent teeth in individuals. Journal of Dental Research. 1957 Feb;36(1):39-47.
12. Bolton WA. Disharmony in tooth size and its relation to the analysis and treatment of malocclusion. The Angle Orthodontist. 1958 Jul;28(3):113-30.
13. Tweed CH. Treatment planning and therapy in the mixed dentition. American Journal of Orthodontics and Dentofacial Orthopedics. 1963 Dec 1;49(12):881-906.
14. Kaplan RG, Smith CC, Kanarek PH. An analysis of three mixed dentition analyses. Journal of dental research. 1977 Nov;56(11):1337-43.
15. INGERVALL BE, LENNARTSSON B. Prediction of breadth of permanent canines and premolars in the mixed dentition. The Angle Orthodontist. 1978 Jan;48(1):62-9.
16. Gardner RB. A comparison of four methods of predicting arch length. American journal of orthodontics. 1979 Apr 1;75(4):387-98.
17. Staley RN, Shelly TH, Martin JF. Prediction of lower canine and premolar widths in the mixed dentition. American journal of orthodontics. 1979 Sep 1;76(3):300-9.

18. Staley RN, Kerber PE. A revision of the Hixon and Oldfather mixed-dentition prediction method. American Journal of Orthodontics and Dentofacial Orthopedics. 1980 Sep 1;78(3):296-302.

19. Frankel HH, Benz EM. Mixed dentition analysis for black Americans. Pediatric Dentistry. 1986 Sep;8(3):226-30.

20. Merrifield LL, Klontz HA, Vaden JL. Differential diagnostic analysis system. American Journal of Orthodontics and Dentofacial Orthopedics. 1994 Dec 1;106(6):641-8.

21. Tollaro I, Baccetti T, Franchi L, Tanasescu CD. Role of posterior transverse interarch discrepancy in Class II, Division 1 malocclusion during the mixed dentition phase. American Journal of Orthodontics and Dentofacial Orthopedics. 1996 Oct 1;110(4):417-22.

22. Davidovitch M, McInnis D, Lindauer SJ. The effects of lip bumper therapy in the mixed dentition. American journal of orthodontics and dentofacial orthopedics. 1997 Jan 1;111(1):52-8.

23. Schirmer UR, Wiltshire WA. Orthodontic probability tables for black patients of African descent: mixed dentition analysis. American journal of orthodontics and dentofacial orthopedics. 1997 Nov 1;112(5):545-51.

24. Lee-Chan S, Jacobson BN, Chwa KH, Jacobson RS. Mixed dentition analysis for Asian-Americans. American journal of orthodontics and dentofacial orthopedics. 1998 Mar 1;113(3):293-9.

25. Ngan P, ALKIRE RG, FIELDS JR HE. Management of space problems in the primary and mixed dentitions. The Journal of the American Dental Association. 1999 Sep 1;130(9):1330-9.

26. Bondarets N, McDonald F. Analysis of the vertical facial form in patients with severe hypodontia. American Journal of Physical Anthropology: The Official Publication of the American Association of Physical Anthropologists. 2000 Feb;111(2):177-84.

27. Wahab Nourallah A, Gesch D, Nabieh Khordaji M, Splieth C. New regression equations for predicting the size of unerupted canines and premolars in a contemporary population. The Angle Orthodontist. 2002 Jun;72(3):216-21.

28. Tootla R, Fayle SA. Comparison of two methods of space prediction in the mixed dentition. Pediatric dentistry. 2003;25(4):350-6.

29. Buwembo W, Luboga S. Moyer's method of mixed dentition analysis: a meta-analysis. African health sciences. 2004;4(1):63-6.

30. Kecik D, Kocadereli I, Saatci I. Evaluation of the treatment changes of functional posterior crossbite in the mixed dentition. American Journal of Orthodontics and Dentofacial Orthopedics. 2007 Feb 1;131(2):202-15.

31. Akcam MO, Toygar TU, Özer L, Özdemir B. Evaluation of 3-dimensional tooth crown size in cleft lip and palate patients. American journal of orthodontics and dentofacial orthopedics. 2008 Jul 1;134(1):85-92.

32. Durgekar SG, Naik V. Evaluation of Moyers mixed dentition analysis in school children. Indian journal of dental research. 2009 Jan 1;20(1):26.

33. Cattaneo C, Butti AC, Bernini S, Biagi R, Salvato A. Comparative evaluation of the group of teeth with the best prediction value in the mixed dentition analysis. Eur J Paediatr Dent. 2010 Mar 1;11(1):23-6.
34. Felício LG, de Oliveira Ruellas AC, Bolognese AM, Sant'Anna EF, de Souza Araújo MT. Mixed dentition analysis: Tomography versus radiographic prediction and measurement. Dental press journal of orthodontics. 2010;15(5):159-65.
35. Philip NI, Prabhakar M, Arora D, Chopra S. Applicability of the Moyers mixed dentition probability tables and new prediction aids for a contemporary population in India. American journal of orthodontics and dentofacial orthopedics. 2010 Sep 1;138(3):339-45.
36. Bherwani AK, Fida M. Development of a prediction equation for the mixed dentition in a Pakistani sample. American journal of orthodontics and dentofacial orthopedics. 2011 Nov 1;140(5):626-32.
37. Butt S, Chaudhry S, JAVED M, Wahid A, EHSAN A, Malik S, KHAN AA. MIXED DENTITION SPACE ANALYSIS: A REVIEW. Pakistan Oral & Dental Journal. 2012 Dec 1;32(3).
38. Khanehmasjedi M, Bassir L. Prediction of the size of unerupted canines and premolars in an Iranian population. Indian Journal of Dental Research. 2013 Jul 1;24(4):493.
39. Galvão MD, Dominguez GC, Tormin ST, Akamine A, Tortamano A, Fantini SM. Applicability of Moyers analysis in mixed dentition: A systematic review. Dental press journal of orthodontics. 2013 Dec;18(6):100-5.

40. Shah S, Bhaskar V, Venkataraghvan K, Choudhary P, Mahadevan G, Trivedi K. Applicability of regression equation using widths of mandibular permanent first molars and incisors as a predictor of widths of mandibular canines and premolars in contemporary Indian population. Journal of Indian Society of Pedodontics and Preventive Dentistry. 2013 Jul 1;31(3):135.
41. Kaur A, Singh R, Mittal S, Sharma S, Bector A, Awasthi S. Evaluation and applicability of Moyers mixed dentition arch analysis in Himachal population. Dental Journal of Advance Studies. 2014 Aug;2(02):096-104.
42. Cruz BS, Rothier EK, Vilella BD, Vilella OD, Nascimento RR. Evaluation of two methods for mixed dentition analysis using the method error. Brazilian Journal of Oral Sciences. 2014 Sep;13(3):163-7.
43. Ramesh N, Reddy MS, Palukunnu B, Shetty B, Puthalath U. Mixed dentition space analysis in Kodava population: A comparison of two methods. Journal of clinical and diagnostic research: JCDR. 2014 Sep;8(9):ZC01.
44. Thimmegowda U, Sarvesh SG, Shashikumar HC, Kanchiswamy LN, Shivananda DH, Prabhakar AC. Validity of Moyers Mixed Dentition Analysis and a New Proposed Regression Equation as a Predictor of Width of Unerupted Canine and Premolars in Children. Journal of clinical and diagnostic research: JCDR. 2015 Aug;9(8):ZC01-6.
45. Hambire CU, Sujan S. Evaluation of validity of Tanaka-Johnston analysis in Mumbai school children. Contemporary clinical dentistry. 2015 Jul;6(3):337.

46. Maroli S, Ali H, Chakkarayan J, Vijayan V, Chinthan G. A Comparative Evaluation of Moyers Mixed Dentition Analysis among Bengali and Keralite Population. Journal of International Oral Health. 2015 Dec 1;7(12):38.
47. Mageet AO. Tooth Size Discrepancy among Different Malocclusion Groups in a Sudanese Sample. Journal of Orthodontics. 2017;3(2):10.
48. F.McDonald, A.J.Ireland: Diagnosis of Orthodontic patient- first edition, published by OUP oxford,1998
49. Graber TM. Orthodonties: Principles and Practice.published by W.B Saunders Company 1966
50. Samir E. Bishara- Textbook of Orthodontics- published by Elsevier 2001 -EDN-1
51. Lloyd ZB. Serial extraction as a treatment procedure. American Journal of Orthodontics and Dentofacial Orthopedics. 1956 Oct 1;42(10):728-39.
52. Barrow GV, White JR. Developmental changes of the maxillary and mandibular dental arches. The Angle Orthodontist. 1952 Jan;22(1):41-6.
53. Lewis SJ. Some aspects of dental arch growth. Journal of the American Dental Association. 1936 Feb 1;23(2):277-96.
54. Carey CW. Diagnosis and case analysis in orthodontics. American Journal of Orthodontics and Dentofacial Orthopedics. 1952 Mar 1;38(3):149-61.
55. Mittal S, Pathak A, Mittal K, Pathania V. Predicting the mesiodistal width of unerupted canine and premolars by using width of the permanent mandibular incisors and first molar in the Himachal population. Journal of Indian Society of Pedodontics and Preventive Dentistry. 2016 Jul 1;34(3):204.

56. Machado LA, Vilella OD, Agostinho LM. Evaluation of two techniques to measure the available space in the mandibular dental arch using the method error. Revista Odonto Ciência. 2012;27(3):228-32.
57. Pawar RO, Bhat SR. Prediction of Mesiodistal Width of the Mandibular Permanent Canines and Premolars by Utilizing the Mesiodistal Width of Mandibular First Permanent Molars and Incisors. International Journal of Scienti fi c Study. 2016 Mar 1;3(12):178-83.
58. Wangpichit K, Huntington NL, Kapala JT. Comparison of three methods of mixed dentition analysis in cleft lip and patients. Pediatric Dentistry. 2001;23(6):478-80.
59. Gramling JF. A cephalometric appraisal of the results of orthodontic treatment on fifty five unsuccessfully corrected difficult Class II malocclusions. Journal of the Charles H. Tweed International Foundation. 1987 Apr;15:112-24.
60. Gramling JF. The probability index. Journal of the Charles H. Tweed International Foundation. 1989 Apr;17:81-93.
61. Merrifield LL, Klontz HA, Vaden JL. Differential diagnostic analysis system. American Journal of Orthodontics and Dentofacial Orthopedics. 1994 Dec 1;106(6):641-8.
62. Horn AJ. Facial height index. American Journal of Orthodontics and Dentofacial Orthopedics. 1992 Aug 1;102(2):180-6.
63. RICHARDSON ME. Development of the lower third molar from 10 to 15 years. The Angle Orthodontist. 1973 Apr;43(2):191-3.
64. Ledyard BC. A study of thę mandibular third molar area. American Journal of Orthodontics. 1953 May 1;39(5):366-73.

65. Lundström A. Intermaxillära tandbreddsförhallanden och tandställningen. Svensk Tandl.-Tidskrift. 1943;36:575.

66. Yuen KK, Lai-king Tang E, Lai-ying So L. mixed dentition analysis for Hong Kong Chinese. The Angle Orthodontist. 1998 Feb;68(1):21-8.

67. Altherr ER, Koroluk LD, Phillips C. Influence of sex and ethnic tooth-size differences on mixed-dentition space analysis. American journal of orthodontics and dentofacial orthopedics. 2007 Sep 1;132(3):332-9.

68. Sonawane S, Bettigiri A, Soni VP. Comparison of two non-radiographic techniques of mixed dentition analysis and evaluation of their applicability for Marathi population. Sci J. 2008;2:1-4.

Kolibri 360 GmbH
Ferdinand-Jühlke-Straße 7
99095 Erfurt, Deutschland
produktsicherheit@kolibri360.de

Druck:
CPI Druckdienstleistungen GmbH
im Auftrag der
Kolibri 360 GmbH
Ferdinand-Jühlke-Str. 7
99095 Erfurt